Seven-Day
SUPER SMOOTHIE
Cleanse
Action Plan

ISBN-13: 978-0692445938
ISBN-10: 0692445935

DISCLAIMER

The information in this book is for your education. It's not intended to diagnose, treat, or cure any medical condition or dispense medical advice. The responsibility for the consequences of the use of any suggestion or procedure described in this book lies not with the author/publisher, but with you. If you decide to follow this cleanse plan, please seek the advice and counsel of a licensed health professional and then use your own judgment.

YOUR FREE BONUS

As a way of saying thank you for your purchase, I'm offering a free recipe book that's exclusive to my readers.

A successful cleanse/detoxification plan can help you remove toxins from your body effectively, sleep better, boost energy, reduce cravings, and lose weight in a short amount of time. The best way to maintain your results or continue losing weight after finishing a cleanse is a healthy lifestyle that involves healthy eating. **That's why I created** *Post Cleanse Meals.* This recipe book encompasses 10 mouth-watering, easy-to-make, healthy recipes that not only satisfy your taste buds but also maintain your weight and health. The majority of the bonus recipes require less than 15 minutes of hands-on time. You can **download this free recipe book here** at http://gourmetpersuasian.com/cleansebonus

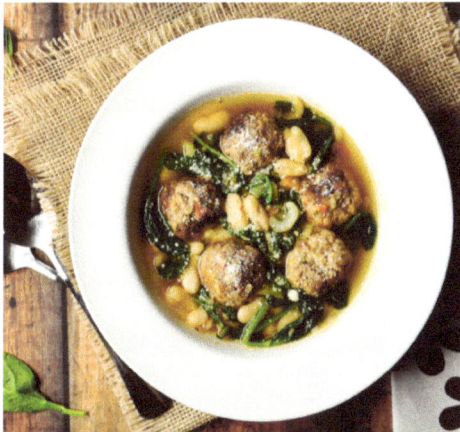

POST CLEANSE MEALS

10 EASY-TO-MAKE MOUTHWATERING MEALS THAT HELP YOU
MAINTAIN YOUR CLEANSE RESULTS AND KEEP LOSING WEIGHT

SHARON CHEN
gourmetpersuasian.com

Table of Contents

ACKNOWLEGEMENT

Thank you to my husband, who helped drink numerous smoothies (including the ones that didn't work out) during the course of the development of this seven-day cleanse plan. And more importantly, thank you for allowing me to be doubtful and whiny, and still encouraging me to finish this book.

I also wish to personally thank Stella Guinto and Amanda Lu for testing the cleanse with me. Without their contributions and support, this book would not have been completed.

DEDICATION

To Stephanie McLarty

Sometimes life could be very unfair.
Unexpected things happen.
But you have been facing your biggest obstacle in life
so bravely and fighting so valiantly to make things better.
It's a tough journey and you are well on your way to the end.
I am so proud of you!

Congratulations on hanging in there through your
heart surgery. I sincerely wish you a full recovery.
And I strongly believe that a beautiful and bright future
is waiting ahead for the beautiful you.

INTRODUCTION

Congratulations!!!

You just took your very first step toward looking awesome and feeling great in just a week!

Let me guess: You have wanted to shed a few pounds, but you hate working out and don't have time for it. Or maybe you received an invitation to a pool party. You say you hate pool parties, but the truth is that you love them, you just don't want to show your body in a bathing suit. Perhaps you have a big event to attend next week and wonder how you can look fantastic in front of the crowd in such a short amount of time. Or, it could be that you are more than willing to go to the gym, but your health condition doesn't allow you to do so.

What if I told you that there's an easy-to-carry-out and delicious way to solve your problems in just a week, without having to even step foot in the gym? *Seven-Day Super Smoothie Cleanse Action Plan* is designed to offer you an easy-to-follow, step-by-step action plan to help you detox your body, lose weight, and, most importantly, build a healthy eating habit by drinking super delicious, super easy-to-make, super healthy smoothies for seven days. If you are worried about being hungry during the process, don't be. Unlike other cleanse plan, there are six nutritious solid meals designed in the plan, such as Spicy Avocado Seared Tuna Combo and Healthy Vegetable Salad with four different dressings of your choice. Why? Because protein from an oily fish like tuna is the key to building lean muscle, and good fats from avocado are sating and packed with omega-3s, which help burn fat and reduce cellular inflammation.

To be honest, I know exactly how it feels to be bloated and have no confidence in how I look. You want a change? Me too! If you don't have to, why go to the smelly gym and get out of breath?

7-DAY SUPER SMOOTHIE CLEANSE ACTION PLAN

Why don't you happily accept that pool invitation and say out loud that you will be there? Regarding that important event next week, how about you focus on picking up the perfect outfit and hairstyle—because you have a plan to look stunning after seven days, a plan that will make your skin glow. And if your doctor doesn't recommend aggressive exercise, why take the risk when you have a better option?

As a dedicated food blogger who strives to encourage people to cook whole foods in a simple and healthy way by creating easy-to-make healthy recipes, I am also a lifetime learner of timesaving methods to eat healthy, stay young, and feel great. My recipes have been featured in *RedBoohk Magazine*, Weather.com, SheKnows.com, Examiner.com, and numerous others. I have created and tested hundreds of smoothie recipes, but only the tastiest and most nutritious ones are included in this action plan book.

Whether you are new to smoothie or know your way around a blender, I'll walk you through the plan day by day, step by step, to ensure that you get the results you want.

- A seven-day calendar with your pre-planned smoothie and salad meals
- A grocery shopping list to guide you through your local grocery store knowing exactly what to pick up, with the exact volume
- A detailed preparation guide helping you mentally and physically prepare for your cleanse
- Exactly what to do and what not to do during the seven days
- Powerful smoothie recipes with clear nutrition facts
- Tips on how to make a perfect smoothie
- Multiple healthy and delicious combo recipes for you to customize your plan
- Vibrant photos showing what your meals will look like
- What to do after you successfully finish your plan
- Introduction to a new lifestyle

7-DAY SUPER SMOOTHIE CLEANSE ACTION PLAN

Corporate professionals, university staff, entrepreneurs, busy moms, and many others who wanted to lose weight and feel great by spending the least amount of time possible have already experienced great success by implementing the seven-day cleanse action plan described in this book.

> *"I lost 2.8 pounds and my waistline was down by one inch after I completed this seven-day cleanse. That's all I wanted! It also broke my craving for unhealthy foods. I never realized healthy smoothies could taste that good!"*
> — Stella Guinto, Real Estate Broker in San Francisco, CA

I promise that if you follow the instructions in this book and make and drink tested smoothies for seven days, you will have your daily recommended vitamins and macro-nutrients in a natural form. By the end of the plan, you will find that you have lost a few pounds, look awesome, and feel confident and healthy about yourself. And if you implement the follow-up steps after you finish the plan, you will benefit from it even more.

This smoothie action plan has been proven to help you lose weight, reduce craving, and eat healthy in just seven days. Whether you want to fit into your favorite jeans again, are hoping to be ready for bikini season this summer, simply need a detox after all that serious eating during the holidays, or just feel like your body could use a cleanse, this book is for you! Action plans won't work without action. Keep reading and start your delicious Seven-Day Super Smoothie Cleanse Action Plan now.

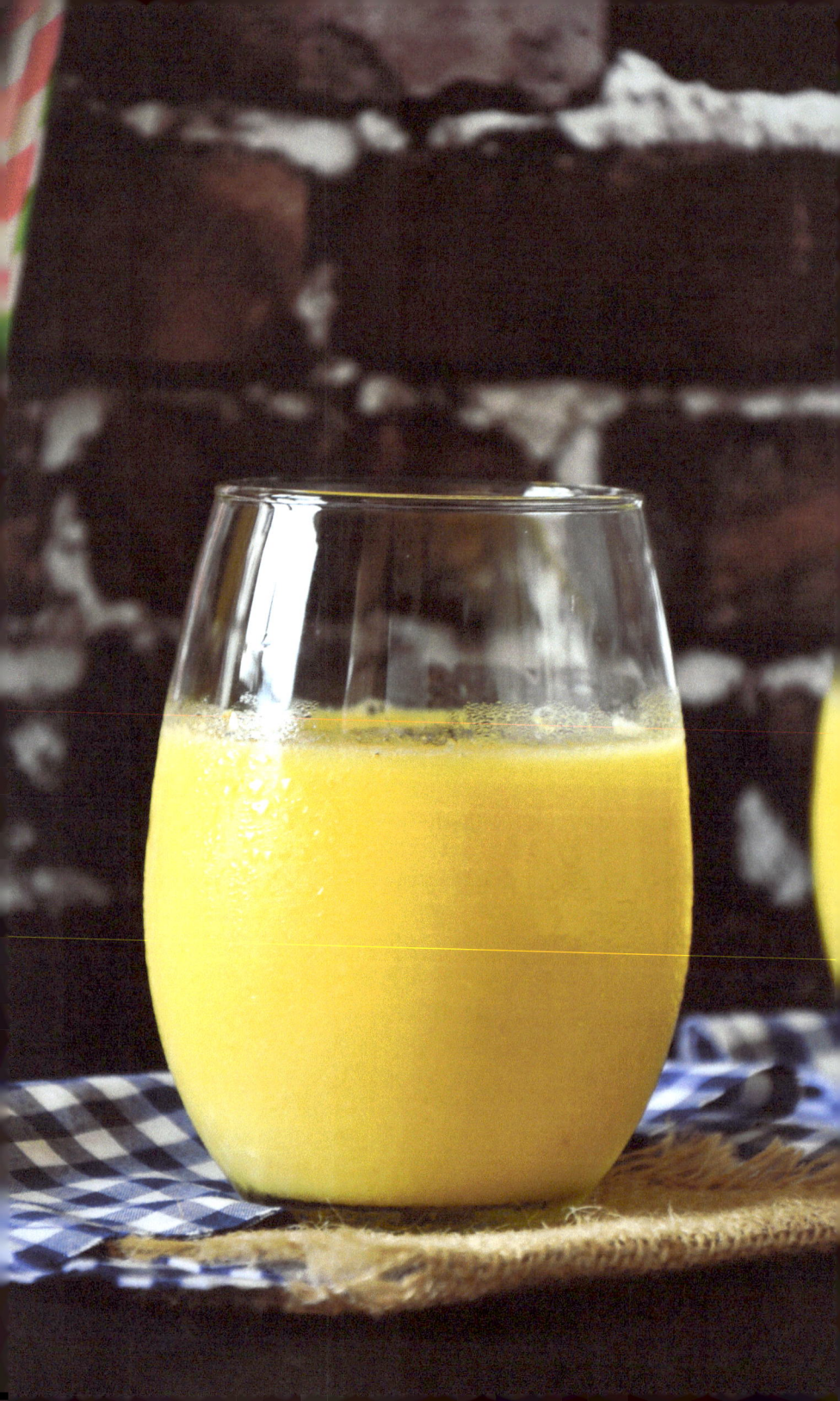

CHAPTER 1

WELCOME TO THE SEVEN-DAY SUPER SMOOTHIE CLEANSE ACTION PLAN

Welcome aboard!

You are ready to make a change—a good one. But you are wondering what exactly this seven-day cleanse is about, and if it's right for you.

In addition to answering your questions right away, this chapter will tell you the best time to clean out your body, and when not to do a cleanse.

In addition, I have a personal motivation for creating this cleanse action plan and I am thrilled to share it with you, because my simple thought at the time turned into this book. I believe it can help you detox your body and, more importantly, help you build a healthy eating habit that can be beneficial for the rest of your life.

WHAT IS THE SEVEN-DAY SUPER SMOOTHIE CLEANSE ACTION PLAN?

The Seven-Day Super Smoothie Cleanse Action Plan is a week-long smoothie-based detox/cleanse with delicious light healthy meals planned in between. The super smoothies in this plan are made of vegetables, fruits, and/or accessible superfoods. They are extremely healthy, and big on flavor too, so you will definitely enjoy drinking them. The light healthy meals are designed to help you ease through the beginning of the plan, as well as the entire process. They also help reduce your cravings for unhealthy food by being delectable. Consider these light meals as a signal sent to your body indicating that you are making some changes, but that they are really good for it. This way, your body appreciates what you are doing instead of fighting against you. After you successfully finish this action plan, expect to drop a few pounds, or to purchase some new pants. And if you kept your old pants, it's time to bust them out because you will be able to slip right back into them. Most importantly, this action plan is going to help boost your energy, change your eating habits, improve your overall health, and get you ready for a brand-new lifestyle.

IS THE SEVEN-DAY SUPER SMOOTHIE CLEANSE ACTION PLAN RIGHT FOR YOU?

You are about to start a long-overdue revolution in your body, but you may be wondering if this action plan is actually for you. To help answer your question, I will break down a few scenarios:

Scenario #1. You've been trying to lose weight, but for some reason you are never really able to do so. For most of us, losing weight is a lifelong battle. It takes time and effort, and, let's be honest here, it's not going to be comfortable. You did everything that people told you to do, such as cutting back on sugars and carbs and exercising as much as possible. You worked so hard to finally lose a few pounds, but you kept gaining them back quickly. It's disappointing and frustrating! Did you do anything wrong? No, you didn't. You just missed an important step—freeing up your body to burn fat.

Your body is smart. It has a built-in mechanism to get rid of toxins through the liver, kidneys, skin, and lungs. Technically, you don't have to do anything—your body's digestive, lymphatic, and circulatory systems do the detox for you. However, all of us are constantly being exposed to toxins in our food, water, and environment, every day. Your body prioritizes removing the chemicals or poisons that are known to have harmful effects on you. Then, if there's still some energy left after fighting for your well-being, your body will work on burning calories. Now, imagine when your body is overloaded with toxins—do you think it will still have the energy to burn calories for you after working extremely hard to detoxify? No. And that results in you gaining weight. But if you could help the amazing system that your body built to effectively and efficiently get rid of the toxins, your body will happily transfer its energy to burning fat for you.

If this is your situation, this cleanse action plan is designed for you to help your body detoxify efficiently. It's a jump start for winning your lifelong battle of weight loss easily.

Scenario #2. You don't have much weight to lose, but you often feel sluggish or tired, or have trouble focusing. Everyone has a unique metabolic system. Some people can eat whatever they want and however much they want without worrying about gaining weight. But that doesn't mean that their bodies are getting rid of toxins on time. Ask yourself: Do you get tired easily? Do you often feel bloated and have digestive problems? Do you have difficulty concentrating? Do you catch colds easily? Do you often have black circles under your eyes? All of these are the symptoms of excess toxins in your body. In other words, not being overweight doesn't mean you don't need a detox.

Scenario #3. You love pool parties but always struggle to show up in your bathing suit. Oh dear! I am totally with you on this one. Knowing that you will be showing off the proud assets of your body and not-so-proud stomach at the same time, you struggle. You look at yourself in the mirror with your bathing suit on. You grab a handful of your love handles and you wish you could just saw it off, saw it off, saw it off…. For the entire party, you control the size of your stomach by trying to breathe in and not let go…. Have you ever done this before? I totally have.

If this is you, the delicious smoothies and foods with protein that are designed in this seven-day cleanse action plan will keep you shedding fat while feeding lean muscle. Muscle is heavier than fat, so you might not lose weight at the end of the cleanse. Instead, you might even gain weight. Don't panic. This cleanse helps you transfer some of your fat into lean muscle so that you will look and feel lean in your swimming suit. After the cleanse, if you continue to eat the food that is recommended in this plan and exercise properly, be prepared to attract some attention at a pool party. Go ahead: Lift your head and act like you own the place!

Scenario #4. You have received an elegantly designed invite to an elegant event, and you wonder how you can look stunning in front of the crowd in a short amount of time. Companies' Christmas parties, friends' wedding ceremonies, grand-opening cocktail parties, conferences…you name it. We all have these important events to go to, and they are great for socializing and meeting new people. Whether you are going to be a host, a speaker, a presenter, a performer, or simply an attendee, you want to be the smart one, and look fantastic under the spotlight, right? Who doesn't?

An effective detox/cleanse can boost serotonin production in the brain. What does that mean in plain English? By increasing serotonin, a naturally occurring chemical in the brain that is responsible, in part, for regulating your brain functions (such as mood, appetite, sleep, and memory), you will enhance your mood and promote better sleep, resulting in a clear mind and glowing skin. In addition, you will also drop a few pounds right before the event. You can do all that through consuming the right simple healthy food for seven days.

Scenario #5. You want to lose weight but exercising is not an option. This might be because you really don't have the time for the gym or you hate working out. It might also be because your health condition doesn't allow you to start exercising just yet. By changing what you eat every day for seven days and introducing a new lifestyle, this cleanse action plan can help you start losing weight right away without working out. However, in order to keep losing weight, you will have to change your eating habits. Also, I will show you how to pick the right type of exercise that you'll love in chapter 6.

WHY DID I CREATE SEVEN-DAY SUPER SMOOTHIE CLEANSE ACTION PLAN?

I'll admit that scenario #5 is a rare case. We are all well aware of how crucial exercise is, in terms of being healthy and staying fit. However, exercising for people like Stephanie McLarty seems to be a little too risky.

Stephanie is the fiancée of my husband's brother, Felix, who resides in Jacksonville, Florida. During time spent in Jacksonville, I got a chance to get to know this sweet couple better. To my surprise, the more I knew about them, the more it broke my heart.

Stephanie was born with a heart problem. She was in the hospital four times in only two months. Each time, her doctor had to shock her in order for her heartbeat to get back to normal. I asked her if she was doing anything special before her heart started beating irregularly. She said she was just in the closet looking for clothes. At that moment, I realized how serious the situation was—we could lose her at any time. On March 24, 2015, Stephanie had her second ablation. (She had her first one in 12th grade.) This time, they also implanted a pacemaker into her body.

Prior to all the craziness, Stephanie showed me a photo of her and Felix taken a few years before she was put on her current heart medication and treatment. She looked a lot slimmer in the photo. She complained about how fast and how much weight she has gained due to the medication. The sad part is that she can't really do normal exercises. She's scared of going to the gym or doing anything that might increase her heartbeat because no one knows when her heart will go crazy again. That's when I started thinking that maybe the best way for someone like Stephanie to lose weight is through detoxifying and changing what she eats every day.

Thankfully, the surgery was very successful. Still, the family has not been ensured that Stephanie's heart is completely fixed, or that there's no further action needed, so it's still necessary to do whatever it takes to minimize the risk.

7-DAY SUPER SMOOTHIE CLEANSE ACTION PLAN

During Stephanie's recovery, I created this seven-day cleanse action plan with the hope of helping her detoxify her body and lose weight. She gladly accepted the challenge. Upon full recovery, she will do the cleanse. I will update you with her results via email. So make sure you sign up for the free bonus recipe book.

WHEN TO IMPLEMENT THIS PLAN

- **When your body needs a cleanse.** How do you know if your body needs to detoxify? The basic symptoms of detox-overload are unexplained fatigue, sluggish elimination, irritated skin, allergies, low-grade infections, puffy eyes or bags under the eyes, bloating, menstrual problems, and mental confusion. Or you may take a detox quiz to find out the answer easily. Take the quiz at: http://gourmetpersuasian.com/detox-quiz/

- **After holidays.** Holidays are wonderful! Thanksgiving, Christmas, New Year's, Super Bowl Sunday, Easter, etc., are all perfect times to sit around the table and spend quality time with the people you love. Holidays usually involve a lot of good food! There's no reason for you not to enjoy your holidays. Just remember to give your body a detox after.

- **Before big events.** As mentioned, a good cleanse can enhance your mood and promote better sleep. It can also help you feel and look great, inside and out, in addition to shedding a few pounds.

- **Before summer.** Got an invite to a pool party? Making plans to hit the beach? Time to do a cleanse for that sexy body.

- **Beginning of the year.** Consider this plan as part of your New Year's resolution.

WHO IS NOT SUGGESTED TO DETOXIFY?

A cleanse is not for everyone. Pregnant women, nursing mothers, children, and patients with chronic degenerative diseases, cancer, tuberculosis, etc., are not suggested to detoxify. If you are training for a marathon, triathlon, or anything that is considered an extreme physical activity, detoxification is not recommended during the time. PLEASE CONSULT YOUR HEALTHCARE PRACTITIONER OR DOCTOR ABOUT WHETHER OR NOT A DETOXIFICATION IS RIGHT FOR YOU.

SUMMARY

In this chapter, you learned what the Seven-Day Super Smoothie Cleanse Action Plan is, and how I started this book. After taking the detox quiz, you know how badly you need a cleanse—and if this one is the right plan for you. (If your quiz score is lower than three, you might already be living a very healthy and toxin-free life. Good for you!)

You know that a cleanse is not for everyone. You've checked with your healthcare practitioner or doctor to ensure that you are free to take this challenge. Great!

In the next chapter, you will see **what kinds of results** you are likely to achieve if you successfully complete the Seven-Day Super Smoothie Cleanse Action Plan, along with a couple **success stories and my personal experience and tips**. Read on.

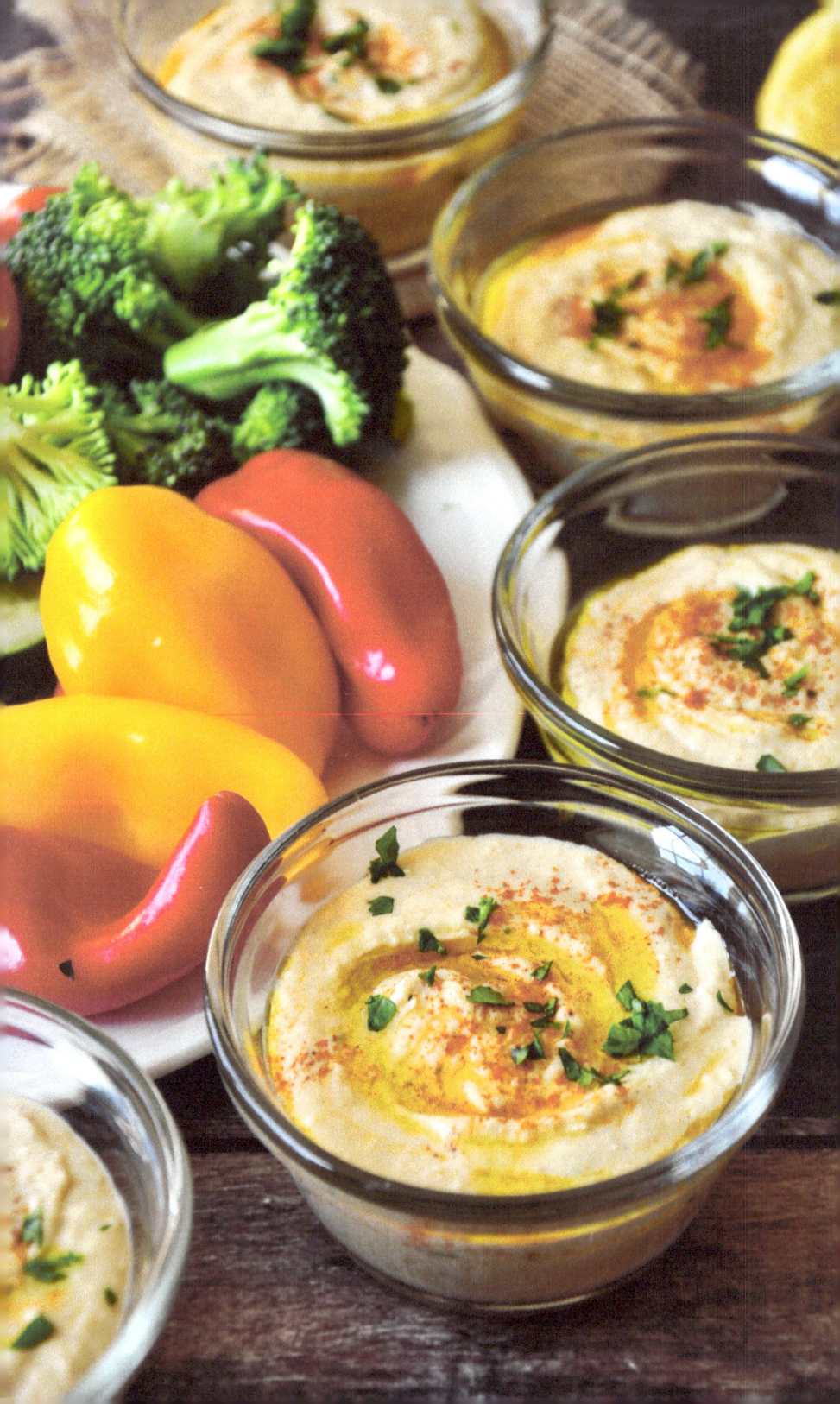

CHAPTER 2

THE RESULTS & SUCCESS STORIES

How well does this plan work? In this chapter, we are going to cover the exciting stuff—what health improvements you can make upon finishing the cleanse, numbers to prove the results, and a few recommendations to help you stick out the plan and get results. I have also included my personal cleanse journal to show you what it's like during the cleanse.

THE RESULTS

After the Seven-Day Super Smoothie Cleanse, expect to see some positive results. The most common health improvements are included in (but not limited to) the list below:

- **Weight Loss.** Expect to lose between three and seven pounds after the cleanse. If you follow the plan religiously, you will drop a couple of pounds by the morning of the second day. Your weight might fluctuate for the rest of the cleanse, but that's perfectly normal. For example, if you work out to build muscle, that will help burn fat all day long. But muscle weighs the most, so some days you might see your weight go up. That's a good thing! If you want to keep losing one or two pounds every week after the cleanse, we will cover how to do that in chapter 8.

- **Pant Size Dropping.** Expect to drop up to two pant sizes after the cleanse. Some people lose pounds, some people drop inches. In most cases, both. Be sure to follow the cleanse journal included in this book to measure yourself and keep track of your progress.

- **Deeper Sleep**. You will notice that your sleep quality improves significantly during and after the cleanse.

- **Mental Clarity.** This usually happens starting from the third or fourth day of the cleanse. You will have a clear mind and greater productivity.

- **Increased Energy**. Energy level is associated with mental clarity. It starts to increase in the middle of the cleanse, and continues to increase over time.

- **Decreased Craving.** You may have thought you were going to have a feast after the cleanse to reward yourself for going through the biggest challenge of your life. The reality is that you probably won't even crave what you thought you would after the cleanse.

THE STORY OF STELLA'S CLEANSE

As a real estate broker in San Francisco, Stella doesn't really have weekends like most of us do. She works long hours every day to serve her local and international clients. There's hardly any down time in her business, so this cleanse was definitely a big challenge for her.

But Stella managed to follow the plan religiously. Her results not only include the number of pounds she was able to lose, but also demonstrate her increased self-esteem by taking this challenge and sticking it out.

She kindly shared her in-depth cleanse journal below.

It was the longest seven days of my life, BUT I have to admit, it was very well worth it! From April 18 to April 24, 2015...

I started at 107.9 lbs and ended at 105.1 lbs = 2.8 lbs lost My stomach was down by one inch, which was honestly all I cared about. I did not want any parts of my body to shrink anymore, as I am on the petite side, with small hips.

Day One - Horrible headaches that made me lie down a lot. I was supposed to work from home, but did not because I was sluggish and headaches would not go away. I stuck with the cleanse and did not eat anything else but smoothies. I hydrated myself by drinking tons of water. Went to the bathroom several times.

Day Two - *As soon as I woke up, the headaches started again, but I was determined to move along and stick with the cleanse. Went to the bathroom several times. Did not lie down to rest, as I had to work the whole day. Had random headaches, but they were tolerable, unlike the first day. Worked from six am until seven pm. Had a teaspoon of pine nuts and had tomatoes for a snack. Had the salad for dinner and shared with my partner. I could not make enough for the next day, as I had a sudden interruption from a client and had to attend to it immediately.*

Day Three - *I decided to go to the gym, as I had not been able to do so last Saturday. At the gym, I looked at my body in the mirror and started liking what I saw. :) No more headaches. I was a little weak at the gym, but I made sure that I had the smoothie before attending my Zumba class. I ate one hard-boiled egg instead of the salad mix as I was starting to really get hungry. Did not have the time in the morning to do my salad mix due to a client emergency.*

I noticed that, due to drinking the smoothies, I felt obliged to hydrate myself by drinking lots of water. I got very thirsty for some reason.

Day Four - *Really good dinner (Spicy Avocado Seared Tuna Combo). I am getting my strength back and do not feel deprived at all.*

I noticed that I am not as tired as the past couple of days. I have been coming home late from work, but I kept awake and did not feel any exhaustion or sluggishness.

Day Five - *I was feeling ok until I got a little hungry at night. I did not get home until 11 pm due to work :(So I was exhausted and hungry when I got home. I still did the strawberry smoothie, but very late, around midnight.*

7-DAY SUPER SMOOTHIE CLEANSE ACTION PLAN

Day Six - Feeling good and getting excited to «graduate." Been snacking on carrots and hummus, and am still committed to my cleanse. It is so hard to stick to a cleanse when you see your partner eating solid food every day. And the smell of his food was almost enough to make me quit and cheat. But I did not!

Day Seven - My last day, and it's Friday! Had two lunch invitations at work but had to decline them. My partner also wanted me to cheat, measure myself already and get on with the normal solid food. "A six-day cleanse is already impressive, so let's go out and have dinner," my partner said. I did it this far, so I decided to suck it all up and wait for the following day to have normal food.

Looking back from days one through six, I noticed that I did not have any issues waking up very early in the morning. Including today, I remained consistent waking up at 5:30am, got my smoothies done, then went straight to my office.

Day Eight - Woke up at 5:30am and weighed myself immediately. A whopping 105.1 lbs!!! I am happy as a clam!!!

I woke up the same time as I did from days one through seven, ready to go to work.

My overall experience: I have always been hesitant to do a cleanse because I do not have a thyroid anymore. I know this Seven-Day Super Smoothie Action Cleanse Plan is not something where you have to starve yourself.

I wanted to challenge myself. I wanted to lose a couple more pounds, and I achieved that. Not everyone knows that I do not eat bananas, hummus and kale. This cleanse has these ingredients. I managed, and now I am used to eating them, all because of the delicious recipes in the cleanse!

Even the day after the cleanse…as soon as I woke up, I made my Crazy Berry Smoothie and brought it to work. This cleanse has seriously changed my eating habits.

7-DAY SUPER SMOOTHIE CLEANSE ACTION PLAN

THE STORY OF AMANDA'S CLEANSE

If you are looking for an example of someone who constantly eats clean food and works out six days a week, Amanda is your role model.

As a certified CPA, no one gets to see her during tax season because she spends crazy hours in her office. Even though she works seven days a week for almost half of the year, Amanda still manages to be the healthiest person among all her friends.

On Saturday, April 25, 10 days after the current tax season ended, Amanda started this cleanse. She hardly had any discomfort throughout the seven days, except for having two bowel movements every day and more flatulence than normal. She attended her intense barre classes five times during the cleanse.

Here's what she says about her experience:

"Honestly, I didn't really expect to lose any weight by doing any cleanse since I work out very frequently. Instead, cleaning my body was my goal. However, I surprisingly lost one pound and 1.25 inched off my waist at the end of the cleanse! Throughout the seven days, my digestion and energy level were significantly improved. It was a great and delicious way to reset and restart my body."

MY PERSONAL EXPERIENCE

Depending upon eating habits and body condition, everyone's experience is going to be different during the cleanse. But the overall purpose and result will be somewhat similar.

I would like to share my personal experience with you, including my results, symptoms that I encountered, how I felt during the seven days, and some personal tips for your reference.

THE NUMBERS THAT MADE ME HAPPY

- **Weight down by three lbs.** by the second day, and it stayed that way throughout the entire cleanse. My weight stopped dropping at 100 lbs. (I am 5'2" tall.)
- **Stomach down by 1.5 inches. Thigh (the biggest part) down by four inches. Lower leg down by one inch and hip down by 0.7 inch.**

SYMPTOMS THAT I ENCOUNTERED

- **Frequent urination.**
- **Headaches.** I am a coffee drinker, so a sudden pause in caffeine consumption caused some headaches at the beginning of the cleanse. The manageable headaches were gone on the third day.
- **Low energy.** The low energy and weakness symptom appeared on the first two days of the cleanse. It disappeared by the morning of the third day, and my energy level kept climbing throughout the rest of the cleanse.

MY CLEANSE JOURNAL

Day One - Went to the bathroom very frequently. Didn't need to snack too much. Had a little headache in the afternoon. Went to sleep at 10:30 pm.

Day Two - Slept very well, but the headache continued in the morning. Productivity and energy level was low. Napped as well as took a bath.

Day Three - Noticed that my sleep quality was excellent. The headache was gone when I woke up. Productivity and energy level increased a lot.

Day Four - Felt totally normal. No symptoms. My energy level went back to 100%, if not better. Took a super smoothie to go.

Walked around the zoo for the whole day without any signs of tiredness or weakness. Snacked on some mandarin oranges and fresh vegetables with hummus in the zoo.

Day Five - Normal. No symptoms. Mind was clear. Productivity was excellent. (I was writing this book.) Took a nap and went to bed at midnight.

Day Six - Completely fine. Did a 45-minute full-body workout and cleaned my house afterwards.

Day Seven - Excited because it was the last day of the cleanse. Yay!

RECOMMENDATIONS AND TIPS

The first two days of the cleanse seemed to be a challenge to me, because my body was adjusting. Starting from the third day, my body was able to get used to all of the changes and eliminate pretty much all the symptoms. My energy and productivity increased significantly. I thought I would crave coffee and pho like crazy. Surprisingly, I didn't. The smoothies designed in this plan were quite enjoyable. They certainly kept my body happy during the cleanse. And in turn, my body rewarded me. Here are a few recommendations and tips that will help you detoxify successfully.

Expect detox symptoms. Done right, detoxification can be very beneficial to your overall health. However, be aware that all cleanses have a number of drawbacks and discomfort involved. There are some common symptoms that you might encounter (especially at the beginning of the cleanse), such as headaches, low energy/weakness, hunger, etc. They don't necessarily happen to everyone, but if they do happen to you, remember that they are completely normal and manageable. We will discuss the side effects and how to manage them in chapter 6.

Focus on creating a healthy eating habit. If you successfully finish this cleanse, you might see the tangible result of a slimmer body. The intangible result, however, is the whole point of this book—

building a healthy eating habit. If you want to do the cleanse so that you can rapidly lose weight, you may achieve your goal. But it's highly possible that you gain that weight back shortly afterwards. Focus on building healthy eating habits. That way, you'll lose more weight and never gain it back.

Customize your cleanse plan. It is important that all the super smoothies and solid food combos taste good so that you enjoy the cleanse and stick it out. Thicken your smoothie with more ice, or add water to make it thinner to your liking. Feel free to add stevia if you would like to sweeten it more. In the appendix of this book, I have included a few more options of both super smoothies and solid food combos for you to choose from. Or, if you discover a few favorite smoothies during the cleanse, repeat the recipes and enjoy them. Feel free to switch things up, but be sure to follow the agenda (in chapter 4)!

Don't starve yourself. The last thing you want to do is starve yourself during the cleanse! This is not one of these starvation diets. Make sure that prepare your snacks. When your body needs to consume more food between super smoothies, feed it with great snacks that are high in protein, such as hard-boiled eggs, hummus with fresh raw vegetables, fruits, and raw unsalted nuts and seeds (only a handful per day).

Take it easy and rest. When you detox, your body is going through a revolution. There will be discomfort along the way, especially at the beginning. You might feel tired or lacking in mental clarity. That's because all the cells in your body are having a big party, getting rid of the toxins they've always wanted dump. Let them have fun—you just rest. It's recommended to pick a slow week to start the cleanse. Make sure you have enough opportunity to rest if you need to.

Let your mind rest too. A detoxification period is a great time to clear the clutter in your mind as well. Try to do some meditation during this period. It will help you relax. If you don't know how to meditate, don't worry—I have covered that in chapter 4. Personally, I found the cleanse to be a good time to get some reading done.

7-DAY SUPER SMOOTHIE CLEANSE ACTION PLAN

Drink lots of water. Drinking water helps to flush out toxins. Ideally, you want to drink eight cups of water (64 ounces) per day. Urination will happen very frequently at this point, but that's a good thing, and totally normal!

Cut down on social activities. Social events involve a lot of temptations, such as alcohol, bites, and desserts that you are not supposed to consume during the cleanse. Besides, if you go out dining with your friends and can't order a normal meal with them, nobody is going to feel comfortable. Chances are that they are going to encourage you to forget about the cleanse, telling you that you don't need it, that you can't do it, or that you should start tomorrow. You have enough negative thoughts on your own. Don't let other people (including your family and friends) add more. If you can find a friend to do the cleanse with you as an accountability buddy, great!! Otherwise, limit your socializing, or only socialize with those who are supportive. Focus on yourself and the cleanse—you will get your reward in seven days.

Keep your cleanse journal. Along with the cleanse, I have created a cleanse journal template for you to easily track your progress every day. You might not lose much weight, but you will drop inches on your stomach, thighs, or hips. Documenting how you feel every day, good or bad, will help you get through the cleanse because the progress is right there in front of you. Even if you cheat a little, no biggie! You are still eating way healthier than you've been eating most days before the cleanse. That's progress. Write it down.

SUMMARY

After reading this chapter, you have a better idea of what it's like to be on this cleanse. You know you will likely lose a few pounds and drop a couple pant sizes, and that you will have better sleep, increased energy, and less cravings. You also know that there will be some side effects at the beginning of the cleanse, and that's totally normal.

But there are so many different types of cleanse plans out there, so **why try this one**? And **what's a super smoothie**?

That's exactly what we are going to talk about in the next chapter. You don't have to empty your wallet to enjoy this cleanse, even though it's enjoyable—especially after the potential detox symptoms are gone. The plan is compiled with delicious, quick and easy smoothies and healthy solid food combos. Even fresh vegetable snacks are made delicious.

Keep reading to find out the reasons and learn more about super smoothies, including their benefits.

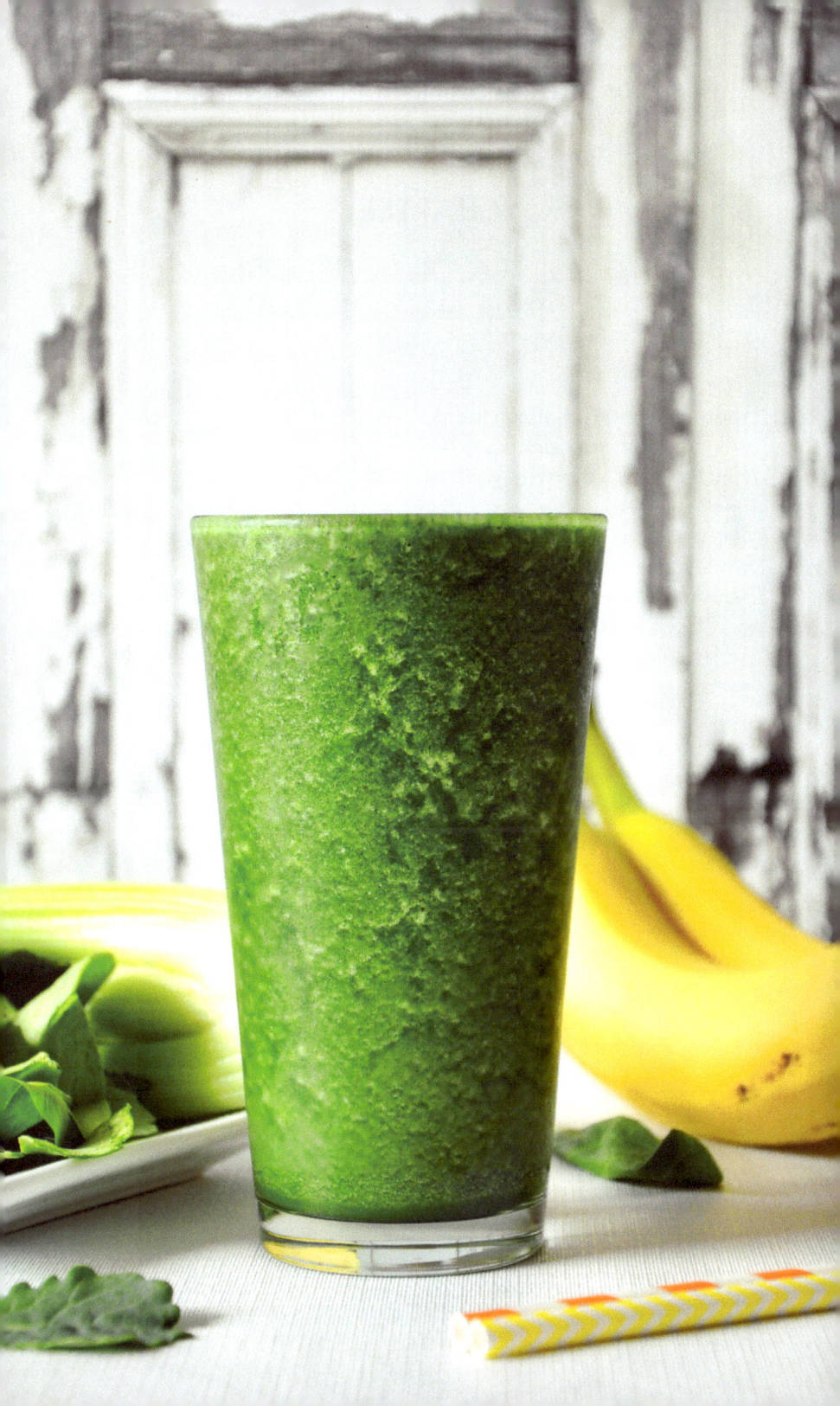

CHAPTER 3

WHY THE SEVEN-DAY SUPER SMOOTHIE CLEANSE ACTION PLAN?

There are many detox/cleanse plans out there. In this chapter, we are going to discuss the difference of this super smoothie cleanse plan, and why you should choose it.

The principle of every cleanse plan is the same: Every once in a while, your body needs a break from fighting toxins (which are now more common in our environment than ever before). If you don't allow this, your body won't give up on you—but it can't make sure to do its best to metabolize the food you eat without excess waste. That's why you have trouble losing weight. Give your body a rest (aka, detox) at least once a year. Clean and nourish your body from the inside out by removing and eliminating toxins, then feeding it with healthy nutrients. Your body will thank you for that. In return, it will protect you from disease, burn fat, and renew your ability to maintain good health.

See, it's not rocket science. Once you understand how your body works, it's much easier to identify when you need a cleanse and why it's so important to your overall health. Now the question is, why the Seven-Day Super Smoothie Cleanse Action Plan, and not others? Before we dive into the implementation of the plan, here is why you are looking at the right cleanse plan.

FOUR REASONS FOR CHOOSING THE SEVEN-DAY SUPER SMOOTHIE CLEANSE ACTION PLAN

INEXPENSIVE

The goal of this plan is to help you understand your body system better, get you through a much-needed detox period by pro-

7-DAY SUPER SMOOTHIE CLEANSE ACTION PLAN

viding you with a step-by-step guide, change your eating habits, reduce your craving, and introduce you to a new healthy lifestyle. **Emptying your wallet is not part of the plan.** All the smoothies, light healthy meals, and snacks designed in this plan are made of mostly common and accessible ingredients. You will see some superfoods included in this plan, but nothing too exotic or pricey. Superfood means super healthy, but it doesn't have to mean super expensive. You will be presented with scientific proof about the ingredients used in this cleanse action plan in chapter 5.

EASY AND QUICK

Unlike most other cleanse plans that outline a ballpark guide to detoxification, leaving you to figure out what food and how much you should eat during each meal to get the protein, fiber, or healthy fat you need to fit into the suggested daily amount, this seven-day cleanse action plan is a system designed to make cleansing easy for you by pre-planning your detox meals, providing you with an easy-to-follow, step-by-step guide (including what to buy at a grocery store and how to prepare your meals), and calculating the daily nutrition amount for you so that you don't have to worry about anything. All the meals are easy to make and very quick to prepare. This action plan only requires you to do one thing—take action!

ENJOYABLE

Let's be honest here. This is not just a smoothie recipe book for you to use as a reference whenever you feel like having a smoothie. This is a book about cleaning your body, your blood, and your mind for straight seven days. Will there be discomfort? Certainly. Any change in life is about pulling yourself out of your comfort zone. However, it doesn't have to be miserable to make a change. New experiences are always going to be different, but they can also be enjoyable. Unlike those no-eating cleanses that leave you hungry and headachy, you will be having solid food during your cleanse. I made sure that every single smoothie or healthy meal designed in this plan is not only going to help you detoxify, but also be so freaking delectable that you will crave them after the plan is finished. And the deliciousness isn't just limited to three meals a day. You will get to snack on any crunchy fruits or non-starchy vegetables you want between smoothie meals. They are a great source of fiber and will keep your metabolism strong, in addition to decreasing hunger. Did I mention that the plan even covers your snack dip? Take action and, more importantly, ENJOY!

CUSTOMIZABLE

This seven-day cleanse action plan is composed with super smoothies and solid food meals (like protein combo and whole-grain salad) for a week. Each category has a recommended recipe, as well as a few more options for you to choose from. For example, if you are not a big fan of tuna, simply switch Spicy Avocado Seared Tuna Combo with Grilled Shrimp Brown Rice Combo or the chicken combo and the scallop combo included in the appendix. The best part of this plan is its variety, allowing you to customize your meals to form your own seven-day cleanse action plan.

WHAT IS A SUPER SMOOTHIE AND WHY?

"OK, this is a cleanse with customizable smoothies and solid food meals. Sounds pretty good. But why smoothie? Why not juice? What exactly is a super smoothie?" you might ask.

Nowadays, whenever people mention smoothies, there is always this giant equal sign between the subject and being healthy. Smoothies have come a long way to establish such a strong and positive healthy impression on us. And they would never have been invented without an electric blender, the only tool that makes smoothies. In other words, the electric blender gave birth to our beloved smoothies. This dates back to 1922. Not everyone owned an electric blender in those days, which is why smoothies didn't become popular until the 1960s, when ice cream vendors and health food stores began selling them. Now that owning a blender is as common as having a cup, everyone can make smoothies at home. How sweet!

However, many of us confuse smoothies with shakes, or even juices. Yes, they are all non-alcoholic drinks, possibly containing fruits and vegetables. Smoothies and shakes even have a very similar consistency. But these three types of drinks are very different in terms of ingredients and health benefits. Here is an easy way to distinguish them.

	SMOOTHIES	SHAKES	JUICES
Ingredients	Contain only natural, non-processed ingredients: liquid base, fruits, yogurt, vegetables, ice	In addition to liquid base, fruits, vegetables, and yogurt, normally contain ice cream, large amount of sugar (like honey), syrup, and other additives	Fruits and vegetables
Nutrition	Fiber, protein, vitamins	Sugar, fat, vitamins	Sugar, vitamins
Required Tool	Blender	Blender	Juicer
Form	Thick puree	Thick puree	Pure extract from fruits and vegetables
Type	Drink/meal	Drink/dessert	Drink

Smoothies vs. Juices

A smoothie typically contains fruits or vegetables in their entirety, as they are held together in a blender—offering the additional health benefits from skin, seeds, membranes, roughage, or other parts left out by juicing. As a result, a smoothie contains all original fiber from fruits or vegetables, whereas a juice only offers extracted liquid. Juicing is more effective for distributing nutrients to people who have limited digestive capabilities or other illnesses. Smoothies are not just healthier, but more filling.

Smoothies vs. Shakes

Oh, come on—let's just face it. With ice cream being a main ingredient, shakes belong on our dessert menu. Smoothies, on the contrary, are considered drinkable meals, with no processed food or added sugar. Which one would you prefer to have EVERY DAY: smoothies or shakes? The answer is pretty obvious.

Allow me to draw a conclusion from this comparison—**a smoothie can be a meal replacement, a shake is a dessert, and a juice is a drink**. In this book, we are going to focus on smoothies as meals and snacks. It's important that we are on the same page about what smoothies are about before we start the cleanse. Knowing the benefits will help you understand more about what you are going to make every day, and help you stick with the plan.

Super Smoothies

People have been making smoothies for almost 100 years, and it doesn't appear that we'll be stopping anytime soon. In fact, smoothies can incorporate additional sources of protein, fiber, iron, calcium, etc. to form balanced meals with macro-nutrients. Superfood supplements tend to be the greatest additional source of extra nutrients, which help us stay healthy, slim, young, and alive longer. All the smoothies in this cleanse plan are made of natural superfoods such as blueberry, spinach, kale, coconut water, etc. Additionally, one recommended superfood supplement like flaxseed, chia seeds, spirulina, or goji berries is incorporated into each smoothie. Those supplements are not mandatory, but are strongly recommended, as they level up your health for a number of reasons.

Let's take flaxseed as an example:

1. **Healthy facts:** Each serving (two tablespoons) provides essential nutrients that we don't easily obtain from normal foods. These include lignans (a type of fiber associated with a reduced risk of both breast and prostate cancer) and omega 3 essential fatty acids (which are essential for health maintenance and disease prevention). Flaxseed is also a good source of iron, zinc, calcium, protein, potassium, magnesium, vitamin E, and folate. Adding ground flaxseed into your daily smoothie will be very beneficial to your overall health.
2. **Economic facts:** Say you buy a 24-oz package of Bob's Red Mill Raw Whole Flaxseed (less than five dollars) and grind at home using a coffee grinder, VitaMix, food processor, or blender. You can make at least 30–35 smoothies with it. Financially, that's only seventeen cents more in the cost of each smoothie. That's a lot of health for a small amount of money.
3. **Flexible facts.** Adding flaxseed to your smoothie provides a slightly nutty flavor, but that's pretty much it. It won't change the main flavor of your smoothie. In other words, you can add flaxseed into any smoothie.

The same facts apply to the other superfood supplements that we use in this book. We will discuss them in greater detail in chapter 5.

SUMMARY

In this chapter we learned that, compared with juice and shakes, smoothies are generally the healthiest way for us to drink vegetables and fruits. Super smoothies are made of natural superfoods and affordable superfood supplements to maximize the health benefits.

We also looked into the four reasons to start this seven-day cleanse plan, which are that it is inexpensive, quick and easy, enjoyable, and, last but not least, customizable.

7-DAY SUPER SMOOTHIE CLEANSE ACTION PLAN

Next we will discuss **how this plan works**, including a **seven-day cleanse agenda** and what to do from day one through day seven. The **YES and NO food list** will tell you what to eat and what not to eat during the cleanse. We are also going to cover **the foods** included in this cleanse in detail in the next chapter. Be prepared to take some **additional steps** in order to make your cleanse successful. Don't worry, there's nothing complicated.

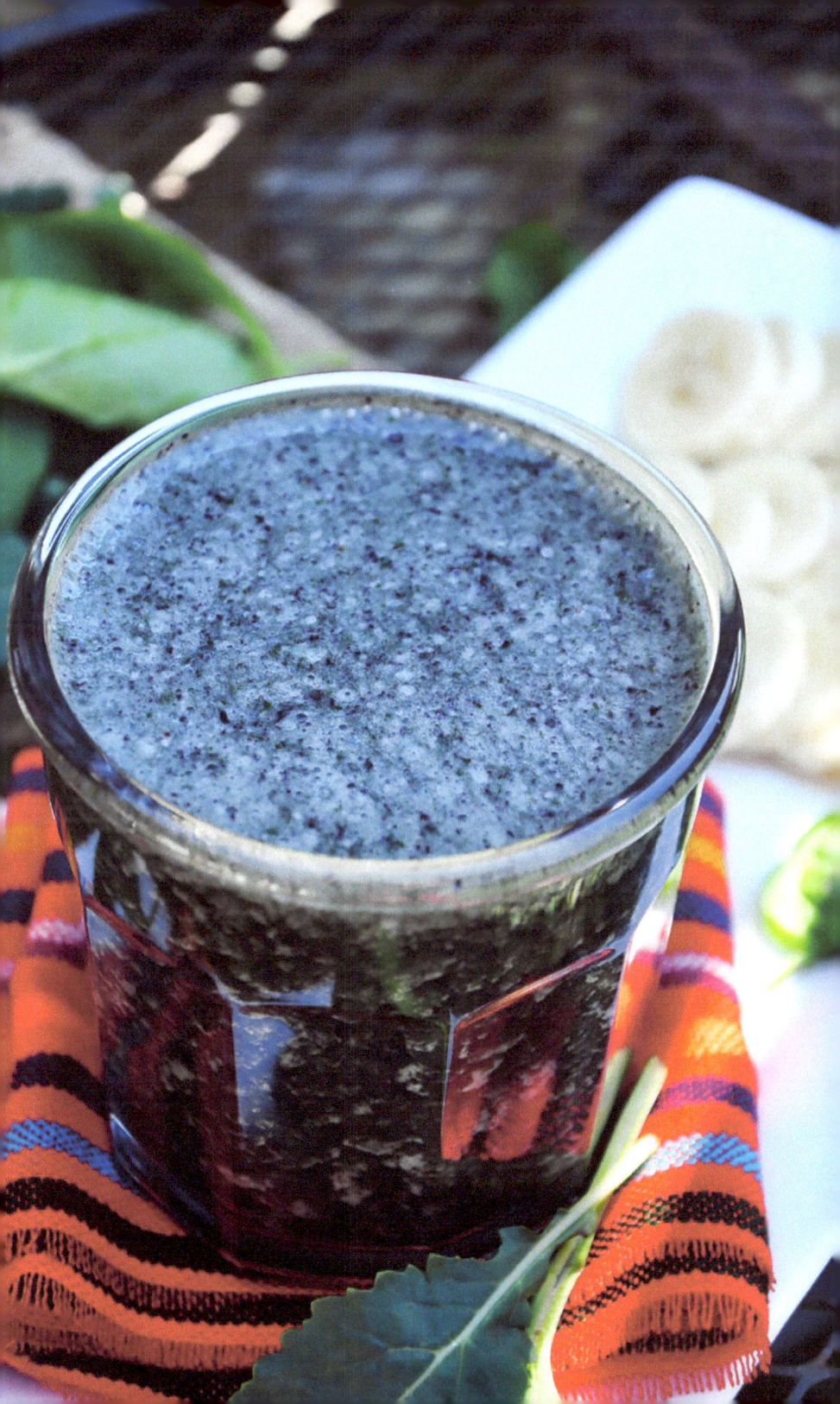

CHAPTER 4
HOW THE PLAN WORKS

2! That's how many pant sizes you will possibly drop after the plan.

3! That's how many pounds you will drop (minimum) after the plan.

7! That's how many days it requires to complete the plan.

21! That's how many meals you are supposed to eat for seven days.

15! That's how many super smoothie meals you are going to have during the seven days.

12! That's how many smoothies you will actually be making.

6! That's how many solid meals you will have during the seven days.

3! That's how many times you will actually make these solid meals.

8! That's how many cups of water you should drink every day, even after the plan.

0.5! That's how many lemons you should squeeze every morning to make lemon water, every single day!

∞! That's how long you will benefit from a healthy eating habit.

You don't have to memorize these numbers. People say that numbers talk, so I went ahead and broke down the whole process into numbers to see if they make any sense to you. I don't know about you, but I am visual learner. Pictures and graphics make the most sense to me. Here is one.

7-DAY SUPER SMOOTHIE CLEANSE ACTION PLAN

THE AGENDA

Day	Measure	Meal	Breakfast	Lunch	Dinner
1	First thing in the morning		Super Smoothie	Super Smoothie	Super Smoothie
2			Super Smoothie	Super Smoothie	Vegetable Salad
3			Super Smoothie	Vegetable Salad	Super Smoothie
4	First thing in the morning	Lemon water before breakfast	Super Smoothie	Super Smoothie	Protein Combo
5			Super Smoothie	Protein Combo	Super Smoothie
6			Super Smoothie	Super Smoothie	Whole Grain Salad
7			Super Smoothie	Whole Grain Salad	Super Smoothie
8	Measure and weigh first thing in the morning to see your results				
Snack	Fruit, 15-20 Raw Almonds, Hard Boiled Eggs, Hummus with Non-Starchy Vegetables: Cucumber, Celery, Carrot, Cherry Tomato, Raddish, Sweet Mini Pepper, Broccoli, etc				
Water	Drink 8 cups of water every day.				

Is this better? Yes?! Good. Let me explain further.

I would recommend you start this plan on a Sunday. Spare your-self enough time to do all the preparation on a Saturday, like picking up groceries, stocking stuff up in the fridge, cutting up vegetables for snack, and such. Allow your body to adjust a little before you go to work.

33

7-DAY SUPER SMOOTHIE CLEANSE ACTION PLAN

DAY ONE

On your first day of the cleanse, you are going to take a temporary break from solid food. You will drop up to two pounds overnight, as your body minimizes bloat and flushes out excess water weight this way. Because it's a Sunday and I assume you don't have to work, you get to enjoy three different super smoothies for breakfast, lunch, and dinner. Each smoothie yields 20 ounces. With protein powder blended in, these smoothies will keep you feeling full all day long. If you can't finish a smoothie all at once, refrigerate it and sip on it when you are hungry.

Did you know that once we reach the age of 30, we naturally lose 1% of our lean muscle every year? The lean muscles are crucial to our metabolic systems when it comes to burning fat. Adding protein powders to your smoothies will not only enhance the flavor and make you feel satisfied, but also help rebuild the lean muscle you need to burn fat.

Another fun task on Sunday is to make the five-minute superfood hummus so that you will have your delicious snack ready for the next six days. It tastes better when refrigerated, and it lasts up to a week or more. Snack when you are hungry. Feel free to make more if you finish the hummus before the cleanse is over. Don't snack all day if you don't have to.

If you have to work on Sunday, pick one smoothie from Day One and make two servings in the morning. Drink one for breakfast and take the other serving with you for lunch. You can enjoy a different smoothie for dinner.

DAY TWO THROUGH DAY SEVEN

From Day Two through Day Seven, you will be eating one healthy solid food meal each day. To make things easier and faster for you, you will only need to cook food on the nights of Day Two, Day Four, and Day Six. (By cooking, I actually mean tossing things up.) The recipes for the Vegetable Salad, the Protein Combo, and the Whole-Grain Salad are for two servings each. In other words, you make dinner as well as your lunch for the next day all at once. Cook three times to make six meals!

On workdays (Days Two, Four, and Six), simply make two servings of the planned smoothie in the morning. If you have a big blender that can easily hold 40 oz. liquid, just double the recipe and blend once. Drink half for breakfast and pack the rest with you for lunch. Keep the smoothie refrigerated. If you have a smaller blender (like the Hamilton Beach Personal Blender that I have), make the planned smoothie twice in the morning.

MEASUREMENT

Before you start the cleanse, take a photo of your entire body and mark it with the date. You are going to take another photo upon completion of the cleanse. That's what we call a "Before and After" shot. You get the idea.

Measure yourself at the beginning, in the middle, and at the end of the cleanse. For some of you, you might not see yourself shedding pounds if you don't have much weight to lose. That doesn't mean that the plan is not working. Remember, the goal is to help your body's elimination system to get rid of overloaded toxins effectively so that it can save energy to burn fat. That's why checking how many inches you are losing is great way to see if you are making progress. Measure your hips, stomach, triceps, thighs, and lower legs the first thing in the morning on Day One, Day Four, and the day after the cleanse (Day Eight). Write down the numbers and document your feelings each day. Do you feel hungry, or cranky? Do you crave all the food that you used to eat? Did you enjoy better sleep? Is your energy level improved? Write down anything that comes to mind. If you cheat, please write that down too, and keep track of your progress. (I won't tell anyone.)

Here's a cleanse journal template designed for you to easily track your progress.

7-DAY SUPER SMOOTHIE CLEANSE ACTION PLAN

Date: Name:

Day 1 Morning	Hip	Stomach	Chest	Biceps	Thigh	Lower Leg
Size						
Weight						
Day 1 Night						
How are you feeling?						

Date:

Day 2 Morning Weight	
Day 2 Night	
How are you feeling?	

Date:

Day 3 Night	
How are you feeling?	

Date:

Day 4 Morning	Hip	Stomach	Chest	Biceps	Thigh	Lower Leg
Size						
Weight						
Day 4 Night						
How are you feeling?						

7-DAY SUPER SMOOTHIE CLEANSE ACTION PLAN

Date:

Day 5 Night	
How are you feeling?	

Date:

Day 6 Night	
How are you feeling?	

Date:

Day 7 Night	
How are you feeling?	

Date:

Day 8 Morning	Hip	Stomach	Chest	Biceps	Thigh	Lower Leg
Size						
Weight						

You may also download the PDF version of the template at:
http://bit.ly/1f2HS4k

THE FOOD

Now, let's talk about the good stuff: the FOOD.

Lemon water. Start off each shiny morning with a cup of lemon water before breakfast. Simply squeeze half of a lemon's juice into a cup of lukewarm water, then drink it up. Lemons help your entire body to flush out more toxins, and prevent built-ups and damage to your cells, tissues, and organs. Lemon water also helps by boosting energy, the immune system, and brainpower, promoting healthy skin, reducing inflammation, and getting you off of caffeine. It's also anti-cancer, and gives you fresh breath. This is something I encourage you to do every day, even after the cleanse. We will discuss the benefits of drinking lemon water every morning in great detail in chapter 8.

Super smoothies. All the smoothies in the plan are made of vegetables (mostly green), fruit, and coconut water, almond milk, and/or fruit juices. Protein powder is usually added in the morning smoothies to reduce your hunger, help build your lean muscles, and provide you with enough energy to get you through the day. Other accessible superfood supplements are recommended in each 20-ounce smoothie, such as flaxseed, chia seeds, goji berries, and spirulina to balance the daily nutrients you consume. Drink a smoothie as a meal. If you can't finish one smoothie at once, refrigerate it and sip on it later as a snack when you are hungry.

Solid food meals. In addition to these nutrient-rich smoothies, the solid food meals designed in this plan are going to gradually ease you into the cleanse, especially for beginners. This is especially great for those who are not looking to dramatically lose a lot of weight in only one week, but simply want to detox and be healthier. The meals also make it easier to stick with the plan and finish it, as opposed to giving up in the middle of it. The six solid food meals are two servings of Vegetable Salad (with four different dressings for you to choose from), two servings of Protein Combo (Spicy Avocado Seared Tuna Salad), and two servings of Whole-Grain Salad (Healthy Quinoa Bowl). Fresh tuna is a great source of protein, as is quinoa, which also offers really good carbs to keep you satisfied. According to the agenda, make two servings of each solid food meal at once. Enjoy one serving as a dinner and pack the other serving as your next day's lunch. We are being efficient and smart about our time!

Water. I can't stress enough how important it is to stay hydrated during the cleanse. Drink at least eight cups of water per day (about 60 oz.), and that doesn't include the lemon water in the morning. As your meals are mostly liquefied, it goes easy on your digestive system. One of the channels for your body to expel toxins is through liquid waste. Dehydration is not something you want to experience, especially during a cleanse. It will cause your blood volume to drop and lead to headaches. Before a meeting, drink a cup of water, and bring another with you into the meeting room. After a meeting, drink a cup of water. After a call, drink a cup of water. When you get back from the restroom, drink a cup of water. If you are bored and have nothing to do, drink a cup of water! In addition to drinking water, you may also drink detox tea if desired.

Snack. Between smoothies you may snack on hard-boiled eggs, fresh non-starchy vegetables like celery, carrots, bell pepper, cucumbers, radish, and cherry tomatoes, or fresh fruit. This plan has made snacking more enjoyable by including a five-minute super delicious hummus recipe that yields two and a half cups. The hummus is made of chickpea, tahini (sesame paste), extra virgin olive oil, lemon juice, and garlic. It adds additional protein to fight hunger cravings and balance your blood sugar levels. Make it on the first day of your cleanse and divide it into five portions (half cup per portion). Only have one portion maximum each day so you don't lose control and eat it all at once.

OTHER STEPS TO THE PLAN

In addition to the eating plan, there are other important steps to make your cleanse successful:

Mind wellness. While you are detoxifying your body, it's also a good time to declutter your mind. Pick a week from your calendar when you can take things slow and easy. Stress will have a negative effect on the body's detoxification systems (including digestive system and immunity), and lead to many other effects on health. The cleanse is a time not only to let your body reset and heal, but also to allow your mind to rest. Try to incorporate meditation into the cleanse. If you don't know how to meditate, **Calm.com** is an excellent tool that guides you to meditate, sleep, and relax from 2 to 20 minutes at a time. Calm also offers a free **Seven Days of Calm** meditation program in their free apps. I highly recommend you incorporate it into your seven-day cleanse. It's a perfect match.

Exercise. Physical activity can get your blood pumping and increase lymph flow and circulation to help sweat out toxins. However, exercising while on the cleanse is a little different from exercising when you are not detoxifying. During the cleanse, although your body will be getting what it needs to be functional, it will also be involved in several processes of healing and renewal. Along with low consumption of calories, it's important to keep in mind that your body is doing a lot internally, so you might not have the energy to stay fully active. Light movement (like 20 minutes of walking, 30 minutes of yoga, or 30 minutes of swimming) every day during the cleanse is good. Remember, listen to your body and take it easy.

Chew. Aim to chew your solid food meal well before swallowing. It can be helpful to bring mindfulness to mealtimes, which improves digestion, allowing you to feel a sense of fullness without the need to overeat.

SUMMARY

In this plan, we start with three super smoothies on day one. Starting from day two, we will have one solid food meal every day for the rest of the cleanse. The solid food recipes designed in this cleanse plan are for two servings—dinner and next day's lunch. During your workdays, simply double a super smoothie recipe and pack one portion with you for lunch. This cleanse plan is designed to save you time and free you from worrying about lunch for the next day.

That's basically how this plan works. To make the cleanse successful and improve the results, try to rest your mind through meditation and do some light exercise to help build muscles to burn fat faster.

The main foods that we are going to consume during the 7 days are 15 super smoothies, 6 solid food combos, and snacks. In addition, make sure to consume eight cups of water each day, and lemon water before breakfast every day.

In the next chapter, we will go further into the **scientific proof** about the ingredients that you will be using during the seven-day cleanse. Some of the most common ingredients might surprise you.

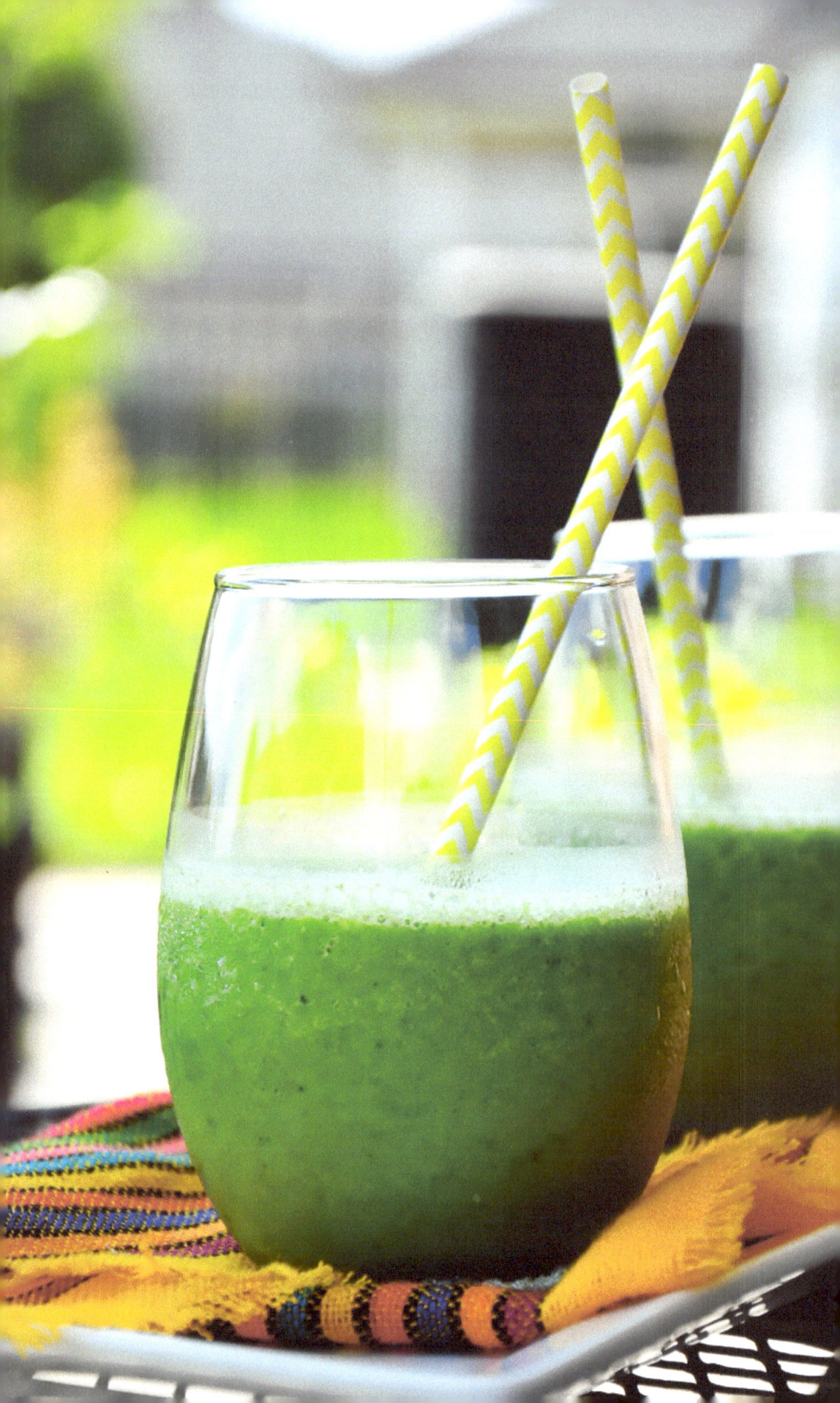

CHAPTER 5
SUPERFOODS FOR
THE CLEANSE

When it comes to superfoods, most of us think that they are exotic and not very accessible. Most of us are wrong! Superfoods are actually just around the corner. Some of them are the most common ingredients that we can get from any grocery store, any day of the week. Many superfoods are included in the Seven-Day Super Smoothie Cleanse Action Plan. Below is a research summary of the health benefits of the main superfoods that are used in this cleanse.

GREEN VEGETABLES

Kale: Deep green kale contains the highest levels of antioxidants of all vegetables, and more calcium and iron than any other vegetable. A single portion has twice the recommended daily amount of vitamin C, which helps the vegetables' high iron content to be absorbed into our bodies. Kale is rich in selenium, which helps fight cancer, and it contains magnesium and vitamin E for a healthy heart. The

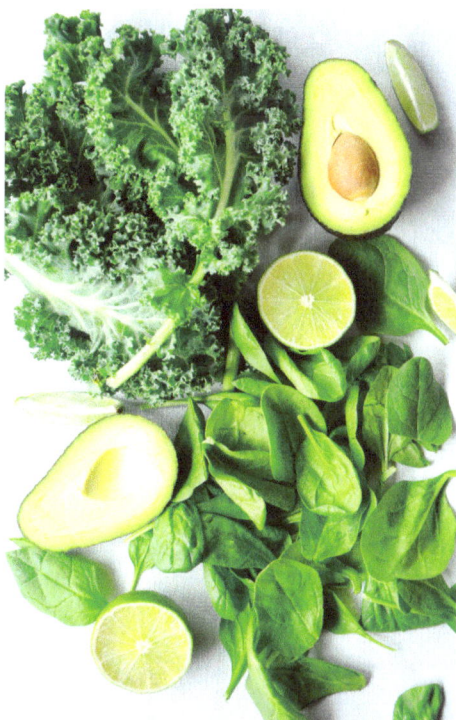

range of nutrients kale provides will keep skin young looking and healthy.

Spinach: Researchers have found that many flavonoid compounds in spinach act as antioxidants and fight against stomach, skin, breast, prostate, and other cancers. Spinach is also extremely high in carotenes, which protect eyesight. It is also particularly rich in vitamin K, which helps to boost bone strength and may help prevent osteoporosis. Its relatively high vitamin E content may help protect the brain from cognitive decline as we age.

Arugula: The leaves are rich in carotenes and are an excellent source of lutein for eye health, including cataracts. The insoles contained in arugula and other brassicas are linked with protection from colon cancer. The leaves also supply a good amount of folate (especially important in pregnancy because it helps protect the fetus) and calcium (for healthy bones and heart).

Celery: High in potassium and calcium, celery helps to reduce fluid retention and prevent high blood pressure. It is also surprisingly high in calcium, vital for healthy bones and nerve function. The darker green stalks and the leaves of celery contain carotenes and more of the minerals and vitamin C than the paler leaves, so don't discard them.

Lettuce: There are dozens of different types of lettuce available in the stores. When choosing, for health reasons it makes sense to pick varieties that are either mid or deep green, or with red tinges. These contain more carotenes and vitamin C than the paler lettuces. Romaine lettuce, for example, contains five times as much vitamin C and more beta-carotene than iceberg lettuce. These more colorful heads will contain good amounts of folate, potassium, and iron. Lettuce is high in fiber, and very low in calories.

Broccoli: There are several varieties, but the darker the color, the more beneficial nutrients broccoli contains. Broccoli is rich in a variety of nutrients that have strong anticancer effects. It is high in calcium, which helps build and protect bones. It also acts as a detoxifier, helping lower "bad" blood cholesterol, boosting the immune system, and protecting against cataracts.

OTHER VEGETABLES

Carrots: The richest in carotenes of all plant foods, carrots are one of the most nutritious root vegetables. They are an excellent source of antioxidant compounds, and the richest vegetable source of carotenes, which reduce the incidence of heart disease, promote good vision, and help maintain healthy lungs. They are also rich in fiber, vitamin C and E, calcium, and potassium.

Red cabbage: A member of the brassica family, purple-red cabbage is high in nutrients and contains protective plant compounds. It is much higher in immunity-boosting carotenes than other cabbages. It is also higher in vitamin C than pale varieties, and is a good source of minerals, including calcium and selenium.

Onions: Did you know that onion is a top health food? The nutrients that onion contains can help protect the heart and circulatory system and may increase "good" blood cholesterol. It is also anti-inflammatory and antibacterial. Onion is very rich in chromium, a trace mineral that helps cells respond to insulin, and is a good source of vitamin C and other trace elements.

Red bell pepper: When green bell peppers are fully ripened, they become red ones. This pigmented red color, along with yellow and orange, contains amazing health benefits. Compared to green bell pepper, red bell pepper has almost 11 times more beta-carotene and 1.5 times more vitamin C. Its carotenoid content is converted into vitamin A by our body, and helps make the immune system stronger to fight in preventing heart problems and cancer. It also promotes healthy skin. Red bell pepper is also low in fat, and is cholesterol-free, thus aiding individuals in losing weight.

FRUITS

Lemon: Being used in many forms, like tea, juice, and even detergents or dishwashing liquids, lemon itself is not only essential to our everyday life, but also has great medicinal and health benefit. Its health benefits are due to its nourishing element contents, such as vitamin C, vitamin B, phosphorus, and proteins and carbohydrates that prevent diabetes, constipation, high blood pressure, fever, indigestion, and many other problems. It even improves our skin, hair, and teeth. Overall, it has great therapeutic properties that are useful for treating kidney stones and the like.

Blueberry: Sweet, juicy blueberries are rich in natural pro-anthocyanin pigment antioxidants. These antioxidants contribute a lot to the optimum health and wellness of a person. Blueberries belong to the family *Ericaceae*, in the genus *Vaccinium*. Blueberries are notable as one of the highest antioxidant fruits. One of the antioxidants contained in blueberry is chlorogenic acid, which lowers blood sugar levels.

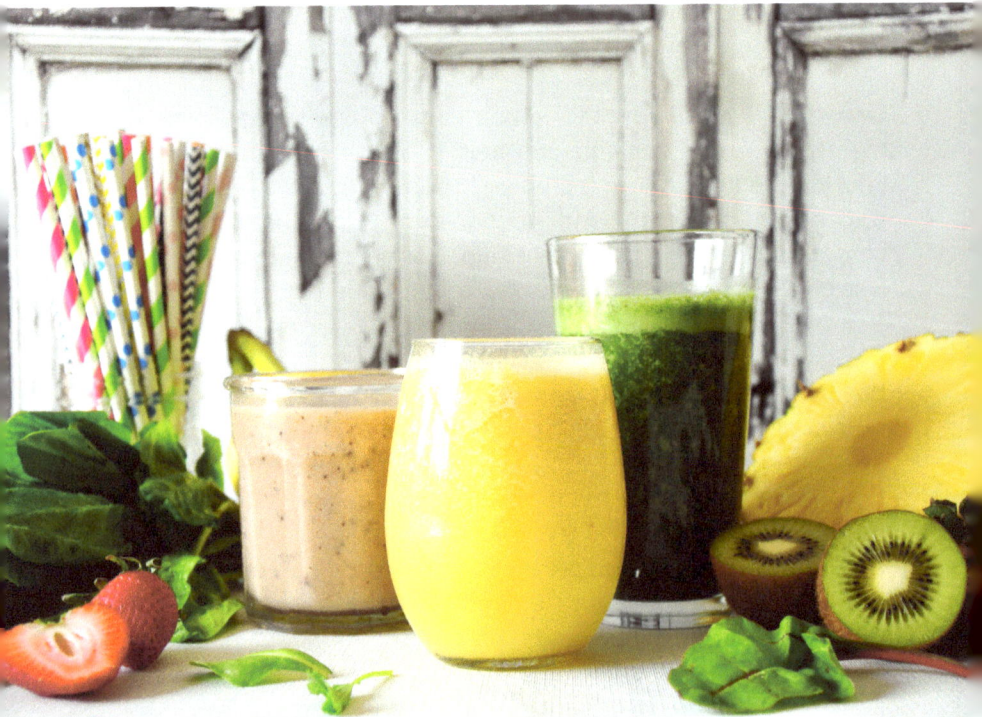

Avocado: Avocado is a pear-shaped berry and is known as a nutrient-dense fruit. Containing nearly 20 vitamins, this fruit is a perfect health choice. Its nutrients are good for disease and infection prevention, especially cancer. It also helps control blood pressure and is good for your eyes.

Strawberry: Strawberries are an excellent source of vitamins C and K, and also provide a good dose of fiber, folic acid, manganese, and potassium. They also contain significant amounts of phytonutrients and flavonoids, which make strawberries bright red. They have been used throughout history in a medicinal context to help with digestive ailments, teeth whitening, and skin irritations.

Kiwi: Kiwifruit is also known as Chinese gooseberry or Macaque peach and is the national fruit of China. A kiwi is rich in vitamin C (containing much more than an orange), is a perfect side dish or appetizer for salad, and can satisfy cravings for sweets. It has also antioxidants that have anti-aging properties. It has many other health and weight loss benefits as well. One great power of the kiwifruit is that eating it will improve the quality of sleep.

Banana: Banana helps you reach your weight-loss goals, keeps your bowels healthy, provides nutrients that regulate heart rhythm, and has vitamin compounds for eye health. Banana contains soluble fiber that makes you feel full as you eat it, and also improves the digestive system. Its potassium content supports normal heartbeat. *Yellow fruits are good for eyesight*, and banana contains vitamin A, which is vital for normal vision.

Peach: With their soft skin and sweet flesh, peaches are a summertime staple. As one of the largest fruit crops grown in the United States, peaches provide a great deal of nutrients with few calories and no fat. Peaches are a healthy way to fit in one of your daily servings of fruit.

Mango: Mango is a tropical tree in many regions of India (as well as other tropical countries) that bears nutritional fruit that can be eaten either ripe (yellow) or when it is still unripe (green). It is called the "king of all fruits" and has many beneficial health effects. Mango fruit is rich in prebiotic dietary fiber, vitamins, minerals, and polyphenolic flavonoid antioxidant compounds. New researched indicates that it is a good breast and colon cancer fighter.

Pineapple: Pineapples are fresh fruits that are loved for their sweet and juicy texture. Aside from being popular for their taste, they are also a great contributor to individual health and wellness. They are loaded with vitamins and minerals that naturally detox our body to fight against diseases and infections. They also strengthen our gums, which hold our teeth. Pineapple is a good cough and cold medicine substitute as well.

SMOOTHIE BASE

Unsweetened almond milk: Unsweetened almond milk is mainly filtered water and almonds. It is a milk substitute from the Medieval European era known for its high protein content. A cup of unflavored, unsweetened almond milk contains 40 calories, 30 of which are from its three and a half grams of fat. It also provides a number of vitamins, including 10 percent of your daily vitamin A, 25 percent of vitamin D, and 50 percent of vitamin E.

Unsweetened soy milk: Soy milk is a rich milk that has numerous nutritional compounds. For those looking for something comparable to dairy, soy milk is the perfect choice. It also contains a large amount of the protein and amino acids needed in a healthy diet. A cup of unsweetened, plain soy milk boasts a calcium content of 299 milligrams, which contributes 30 percent toward your recommended daily calcium intake. The iron in soy milk helps your red blood vessels function properly, ensuring that all the tissues throughout your body get the oxygen they need.

Coconut Water: Coconut water is composed of many naturally occurring bioactive enzymes such as acid phosphatase, catalase, dehydrogenase, diastase, peroxidase, RNA-polymerases, etc. In effect, these enzymes help with digestion and metabolism. Despite being very light in consistency, coconut water proportionately has a better composition of minerals like calcium, iron, manganese, magnesium, and zinc than some of the fruit juices (such as orange).

SUPERFOOD POWDERS & SEEDS

Flaxseed: Flaxseed is one of the most concentrated plant sources of omega 3 fats. Flaxseed contains 50 to 60 percent omega 3 fatty acids in the form of alpha linolenic acid. It is also rich in antioxidants, B vitamins, dietary fiber, a group of phytoestrogens called lignans, protein, and potassium. These tiny little seeds boost your metabolism. Experts advise a ground preparation rather than whole seeds for easier digestion. It is highly beneficial for heart health.

Chia seeds: Chia seeds are known as a great plant-based source of omega 3 fatty acids, in addition to a host of other nutrients. They also have an abundance of calcium, protein, and fiber. Their high omega 3, calcium, boron, and antioxidant content can help create healthy, moist, disease-free skin.

Spirulina: Spirulina is an herb. Just like any other plant, it contains chlorophyll that is absorbed from the sun. Spirulina is a natural powder that is incredibly high in protein and a good source of antioxidants, B vitamins and other nutrients. Many people promote spirulina as a treatment for a range of metabolic and heart health issues, including weight loss, diabetes, and high cholesterol (according to the National Institutes of Health [NIH]). As an antioxidant, spirulina helps combat cell and DNA damage, thus helping to prevent cancer, heart diseases, etc.

Goji berries: Goji berries are known as the most nutritionally dense fruit in existence. Although they have only been introduced in Western countries in recent years, gojis have been used for thousands of years in Tibet and China, both as a culinary ingredient and medicinally. They are also known as "wolfberries" and have many health benefits. They are high in antioxidants, help prevent vision loss, improve male fertility, and are high in nutrients.

Cocoa powder: Chocolates are being avoided due to their sugar content, which can cause many kinds of diseases—but not cocoa powder! In fact, cocoa powder, which comes from the cocoa bean, is highly nutritious and can provide numerous health benefits. Most notably, cocoa demonstrates significant benefits for the cardiovascular system, helping to reduce the risk of heart attack and stroke, high blood pressure, and even cancer.

SOLID FOOD CHOICE

Chickpea: Often called garbanzo beans, these very versatile legumes are commonly served in salads or as toasted snacks. Chickpeas contain vitamin K, folate, phosphorus, zinc, copper, manganese, choline, and selenium. In addition to being an excellent vegan and gluten-free source of protein and fiber, chickpeas also contain exceptional levels of iron, vitamin B6, and magnesium. They have a wide variety of health benefits, such as contributing to weight loss, energy production, protein for vegetarians, contributing to hormone production, etc.

Tahini: Tahini (also known as sesame butter or sesame paste) consists of sesame seeds that are blended with just enough vegetable oil to produce a paste-like consistency. Tahini is quite versatile, and is worth using in other dishes because it packs a big nutritional punch. There are many reasons why sesame seeds are essential to a healthy diet, and have even been called the "lifesaver" seed. They have healthy omega 3 and omega 6 fatty acids, which are good for our brains and hearts, helping to prevent any heart- or brain-related diseases. Tahini health benefits include four important nutrients that provide support to your immune system—namely copper, zinc, selenium, and iron. They are also a great source of antioxidants.

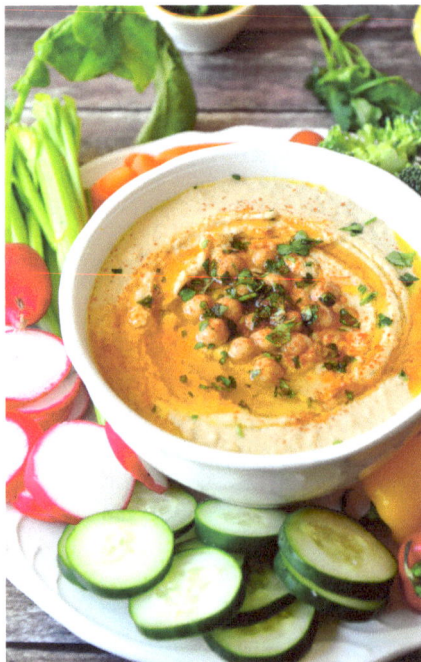

Quinoa: Scientists agree that quinoa is a superfood. It is not just a grain, but a healthy beneficial seed as well. Quinoa is naturally gluten-free and contains iron, B vitamins, magnesium, phosphorus, potassium, calcium, vitamin E, and fiber. It is one of the most complete foods in nature, containing almost all of the needed vitamins and minerals for our daily intake. Consuming adequate amounts of whole-grain quinoa reduces the risk of heart-related problems, high blood pressure, colon cancer, and even obesity.

Tuna: Experts and researchers found tuna to be the "new health food" for its beneficial contents. Having omega 3 properties and the mineral selenium, tuna fish gives us the antioxidant protection that the minerals themselves provide to the fish. In addition, selenium helps in lowering the risk of mercury-related problems, so there is no need to worry about the mercury content of tuna. This healthy food protects our hearts from many types of diseases, boosts our brain cells, and improves our immune systems.

OTHER

Olive Oil: Olive oil has countless benefits. One great contribution of virgin olive oil is the way it improves our health. Despite its high fat content, olive oil has MUFAs, which are considered to be healthy dietary fat. It is a good oil that helps us fight against both types of diabetes, coronary disease, and numerous other diseases.

Stevia: Stevia is a 100% natural, zero calorie sweetener with a number of health benefits that have been confirmed in human studies. And unlike other sugar substitutes, stevia comes from a plant. Stevia has different sweet compounds, one of which is stevioside, which lowers blood pressure. It also lowers blood sugar, which can help treat diabetes. Recent studies even noted that stevia is beneficial to the health of our pets/animals.

SUMMARY

The superfoods listed in this chapter are what we will be blending, handling, and cooking during this seven-day cleanse. Use this chapter as a reminder or a reference, even after the cleanse. Know your food and how it's going to help your body get healthy.

Now that you know a lot about the plan, including how it works, what it's like, and even the detailed food contained in this plan, it's time to roll up your sleeves and get ready for this special week. In the next chapter, I will show you how to get both **mentally** and **physically** prepared for the cleanse.

Here is what we will cover in the next chapter:

- The most common **detox side effects** and how to deal with them if they happen to you.
- A **cleanse calendar** that displays the actual meals you will be eating.
- A **Yes/No food list** that tells you what food is welcome and what food to avoid during the cleanse.
- A print-friendly **grocery shopping list** provided for your convenience.
- **Useful tips** to show you how to make a perfect smoothie.

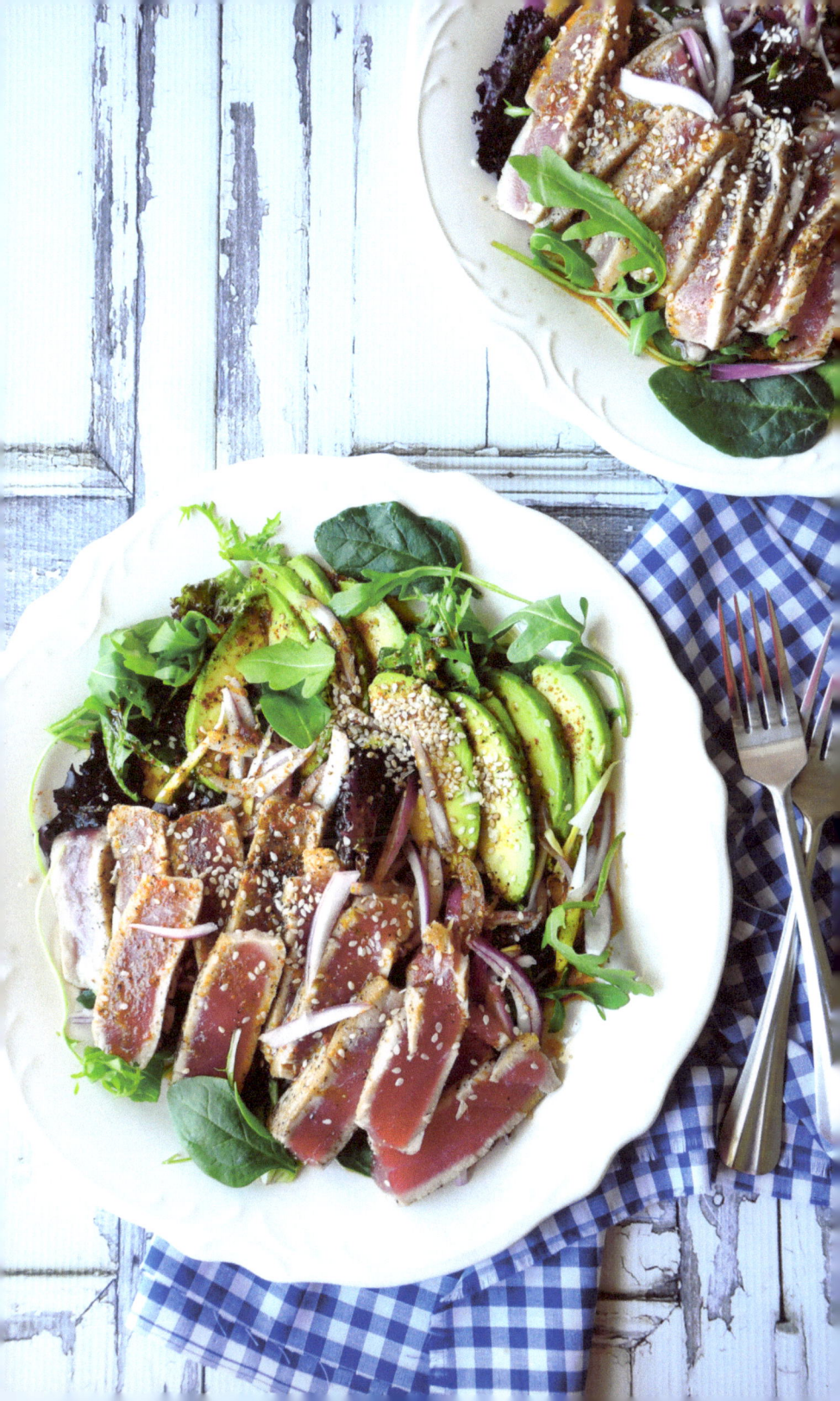

CHAPTER 6

GETTING PREPARED

By now, you have learned about your body, the basics of this cleanse, how this plan works, and how it can help you. Now let's get you prepared for the action. First thing you should know is that there are side effects, especially for first timers. Because you are making some big changes that your body has never experienced before, expect it to have certain reactions. Even stopping doing the things you normally do for a few days (like drinking coffee, soda, or alcohol, eating refined sugar, or smoking cigarettes) will trigger such reactions, not to mention that you will be consuming mostly raw foods instead of cooked foods, which is what most of us are used to.

SIDE EFFECTS AND HOW TO MANAGE THE SYMPTOMS

Some of the most common cleanse symptoms include headaches, body aches, skin rashes, hunger and craving, bowel disturbance, frequent urination, persistent flatulence, and fatigue. **Keep in mind that not everyone is going to encounter the same side effects. Not all the side effects are going to happen to you.** It largely depends on your body conditions. If you happen to have any of these symptoms, remember that they are normal during a cleanse. It also indicates that you are making progress. In this chapter, we are going to learn why the side effects occur, and how to be proactive in supporting your body's ability to cleanse itself through its inherent toxin elimination system.

Symptom #1 Bowel Disturbance and Frequent Urination

Let's start with the most common side effect of detox. Since the mass majority of the food you will be having during the cleanse is in liquid form, the process directly affects the digestive system. By detoxifying, you are being proactive about cleansing yourself. During this time, the cells of your body suddenly have an opportunity to release an even greater than normal amount of toxins, and everything else that is potentially a health hazard—which triggers frequent or even uncomfortable bowel movements, especially at the beginning of the cleanse. As toxins are also expelled via liquid waste, you will experience frequent urination as well.

How to Manage

It is extremely important to stay hydrated during the whole cleansing process. As your body will be excreting lots of liquid, drinking a great amount of water every day is highly recommended. This will also help reduce headaches during the cleanse.

Symptom #2 Headaches and Body Aches

Although a clear cause for this particular symptom during detoxification process hasn't been identified, frequent urination leads to potential dehydration, and dehydration causes your blood volume to drop, which lowers the flow of blood and oxygen to the brain, leading to headaches. That's why you want to be sure to properly hydrate. If you normally drink a lot coffee, the possibility of experiencing headaches is going to be higher.

Temporary headaches and pains within the first couple of days of your cleanse may also be psychological in nature. When you undergo a revolution like detoxification of your body, you become extra aware of its reactions. All of a sudden, these minor pains and aches stand out and get noticed when you are doing something that's supposed to fix your body.

How to Manage

There are several ways to remedy headaches, other than staying hydrated. One is through massage therapy to improve the blood flow in the brain, which eases pain and tension. Placing wrapped ice cubes on the painful area for 10–15 minutes will also help to reduce the swollen vessels that are pressing on the nerves and sending pain messages to the brain. It's not recommended to take anything for the headache, as this might disrupt the cleanse or cause more discomfort.

Body aches and joint pains can be reduced through a hot Epsom salt bath. According to nutritionist Dr. Hazel Parcells, hot water helps draw toxins to the surface of the skin. As the water cools down, the toxins are pulled into the cooled water via the principle of osmosis. While hot baths keep your elimination channels open and gently encourage the detoxification process on a regular basis, according to the Epsom Salt Industry Council, adding two cups of Epsom salts to your bathtub and soaking for 20–30 minutes helps ease muscle pain, lower blood pressure, and eliminate harmful substances from the body.

Symptom #3 Hunger and Cravings

Most people think a cleanse or detox equals starvation. Hunger is by far the most difficult side effect to deal with in many strict no-eating cleanses, because it can cause other symptoms such as irritability. Not eating some of your favorite foods will make you angry easily, so you might want to give people around you a heads up if you feel cranky. At the beginning of the cleanse, your body craves food that it used to consume (such as meat, dairy, sugar, caffeine, etc.) as your body struggles to adjust to the absence of this food and solid food in general.

How to Manage

Don't starve yourself. Drink lemon water, sip on smoothies, have a piece of fruit, a hard-boiled egg, or snack on non-starchy vegetables like celery, carrot, radish, cucumber, etc. when you are hungry. In this plan, a five-minute hummus made with only superfoods will increase the joy of snacking on those raw vegetables. However, if you snack all day, you are not going to lose any weight. The feeling of hunger will eventually decrease significantly as your body acclimates and gets rid of overloaded toxins.

Symptom #4 Fatigue, Weakness and Low Energy

These are very common side effects, especially in most intensive cleanses where calories are significantly lacking. Your body gets energy from calories, which come from three sources: fats, proteins, and carbohydrates. A detoxification will easily drain you if none of these sources are taken into account.

How to Manage

This cleanse plan is designed to have a proper amount of natural fats and proteins to decrease these symptoms. The best way to deal with low energy during a cleanse is to avoid physical labor and exercise. Don't attempt to work out or engage in any strenuous activities. Just rest and take it easy.

Symptom #5 Skin Rashes

If you experience skin breakouts during a cleanse, it means that your body is eliminating toxins through your largest organ—your skin.

How to Manage

A detox bath with salt or essential oil will help reduce the skin breakouts and rashes. Brushing the skin of the entire body while it's dry with a nature bristle skin brush is a fantastic method both for minimizing skin rashes and stimulating and supporting your body in excreting toxins.

The health benefits and increased energy that can be derived from the process of this cleanse action plan are very much worth the effort. However, be aware that all cleanses have a number of drawbacks and discomfort involved. Again, not everyone will have the same symptoms. But when it does happen to you, remember that it's completely normal and totally manageable.

7-DAY SUPER SMOOTHIE CLEANSE ACTION PLAN

THE CALENDAR

Here's exactly what to expect during the seven-day cleanse:

Day	Measure	Meal	Breakfast	Lunch	Dinner
1	First thing in the morning		Goji Green	Ginger Mango	Avocado Pineapple
2			Super Power	Super Power	Vegetable Salad
3			Avocado Cucumber	Vegetable Salad	Classic Berry
4	First thing in the morning	Lemon water before breakfast	Green Lover	Green Lover	Spicy Avocado Seared Tuna
5			Chocolate Banana	Spicy Avocado Seared Tuna	Kiwi Strawberry
6			Peachy Greens	Peachy Greens	Healthy Quinoa Bowl
7			Crazy Berries	Healthy Quinoa Bowl	Cinnamon Peach
8	Measure and weigh first thing in the morning to see your results				
Snack	Fruit, 15-20 Raw Almonds, Hard Boiled Eggs, Hummus with Non-Starchy Vegetables: Cucumber, Celery, Carrot, Cherry Tomato, Raddish, Sweet Mini Pepper, Broccoli, etc				
Water	Drink 8 cups of water every day.				

58

THE YES/NO FOOD LISTS

Before diving into the core of the plan, let me set things straight. You are on a cleanse, so eating whatever you like is no longer an option during these seven days. This plan is not the strictest one on the planet (it's actually quite the opposite), but we do have a few restrictions. Here is a list of the foods you **can** and **cannot** eat during the cleanse.

The YES Food List

Fruit: Crunchy fruits. (Please go easy on fruit, as there are plenty of fruits in the super smoothies already. Too much fruit will spike your blood sugar, cause headaches, and give you an odd feeling under your skin.)
Vegetables: Non-starchy fresh vegetables like cucumber, celery, carrot, bell pepper, radish, cherry tomato, etc.
Oils: Olive oil (preferably extra virgin), coconut oil (unprocessed).
Nuts: Raw, unsalted almonds, walnuts, macadamias, and cashews.
Eggs: Hard-boiled eggs.
Seeds: Raw, unsalted sesame, pumpkin, and sunflower seeds.
Tea: Green tea, white tea, or other herbal tea.
Water: At least eight cups per day, detox water.

The NO Food List

Coffee
Alcohol
Cigarettes
Refined sugar, honey, maple syrup, artificial sweeteners
Cheese
Milk products (except half cup Greek plain yogurt per day)
Meat
Sodas/diet sodas
Processed foods
Fried foods
Refined carbs (white bread, donuts, pastas, etc.)

Grocery Shopping List

FRESH FRUIT

8 lemons
2 limes
2 kiwifruits (not too ripe, since we are going to save them for day five)

9 medium-sized ripe bananas (don't worry about them going bad—you are going to freeze 7 of them when you get home)

FRESH VEGETABLES

2 small red onions
2 avocados (not too ripe)
1 (12-oz) bag spring mix (spinach, arugula, cabbage, etc.)
1 (12-oz) bags kale and spinach mix or other green mix (pick up more if needed on day four when you go buy the fresh tuna)

1 large red bell pepper (half for snack)
1 (9-oz) package broccoli florets
1 (10-oz) bag carrot matchsticks
2–3 medium-sized cucumbers
1 package celery
1 head lettuce, any kind
1 small head red cabbage

1 small package sweet mini peppers (for snack, optional)
1 bunch radish (for snack, optional)
1 package cherry tomatoes (for snack, optional)
1 (12-oz) bag baby carrots (for snack, optional)

HERBS

1 bunch cilantro
1 fresh head ginger
1 bunch green onion

1 head garlic
1 small bunch parsley (for garnishing the hummus, optional)

7-DAY SUPER SMOOTHIE CLEANSE ACTION PLAN

FROZEN VEGETABLES AND FRUITS

1 (10.8-oz) bag mixed vegetables
(carrots, peas, green beans)
1 (12- to 16-oz) bag frozen pineapple
1 (12- to 16-oz) bag frozen blueberries

1 (12- to 16-oz) bag frozen berry mix
(raspberries, blueberries, and
blackberries)
1 (12- to 16-oz) bag frozen mango
1 (12- to 16-oz) bag frozen strawberries
1 (12- to 16-oz) bag frozen peaches

P.S. The frozen fruits listed above are enough for completing this cleanse. I would recommend that you pick up large bags of frozen fruit, as they are cheaper and you can easily store them in your freezer for later. Together with drinking lemon water every morning, drinking smoothies for breakfast every day is something I would suggest you in the long term.

SMOOTHIE LIQUID BASE

1 liter unsweetened coconut water
Half gallon orange juice

Half gallon original almond milk or half
gallon original soy milk
1 lb. Greek plain yogurt

SUPERFOOD SUPPLEMENT

(Optional but highly recommended!)

Protein powder, vanilla flavored
Spirulina
Ground flaxseed (you may buy whole
seeds and grind in a coffee grinder)

Chia seeds
Goji berries

P.S. It's totally okay if you decide not to add any superfood supplements to your smoothies. But I would strongly recommend you pick up some vanilla-flavored protein powder. Many morning smoothie recipes designed in this plan have protein powder in them. It helps give you energy, decreases your hunger, builds muscles, and enhances the smoothies' flavor. I often store a 5-pound bottle at home. You may find all of these superfoods in a grocery store like Whole Foods Market. In the list above, I have

7-DAY SUPER SMOOTHIE CLEANSE ACTION PLAN

included Amazon links to 2-pound bottles of protein powder and 16-oz bottles of spirulina (smaller sizes are available as well) that I personally use, in case you can't find them in the grocery store.

OTHER

1 (15-oz) can chickpeas
1 (8-oz) package quinoa
1 (15-oz) can tahini (or less—you'll need at least 1/2 cup)
8 oz. fresh tuna steak (I recommend to pick it up on day four to ensure the freshness)

Raw almonds (for snack, optional)
1 package cocoa powder
1 (40-packet) box stevia
1 (12-count) package eggs (make hard-boiled eggs for snack)

FROM YOUR OWN PANTRY

Extra virgin olive oil
Sea salt
Ground black pepper
Dijon mustard
Paprika (for garnishing the hummus, optional)

Cayenne pepper
Soy sauce
White sesame seeds
Dried basil
Ground cinnamon

P.S. If any of these items are missing from your pantry, remember to grab some when you are in the grocery store.

You can download the print-friendly grocery shopping list at: http://bit.ly/1MInwZi

PREPARATION

After getting all the ingredients, you want to peel seven bananas, place them into one or several Ziploc bags, and freeze them. They will come in very handy when making smoothies. That's pretty much it. There is really not that much to prepare physically, considering you will be having mostly raw foods for the next seven days.

Keep your cleanse journal template handy so that you can easily reach it every day to document your progress and results.

TIPS FOR MAKING A PERFECT SMOOTHIE

Smoothies are probably the easiest meal you can make at home. We often see a one-sentence instruction in a smoothie recipe, which is "place all ingredients into a blender and blend until smooth." Technically, that's absolutely true, especially if you own a high-end blender with a very powerful motor. However, placing smoothie ingredients into your blender in a certain order can not only ensure that your blender works efficiently and protect the motor, but also save you significant preparation and blending time.

How to Make a Perfect Smoothie

The order that I am about to show you is a detailed breakdown instruction for making a perfect smoothie that applies to all smoothies, including the ones in this cleanse. Once you've learned what goes into your blender first and what goes in it later, making smoothies is going to be a breeze.

7-DAY SUPER SMOOTHIE CLEANSE ACTION PLAN

5. 2-4 Tbsps protein powder, cocoa powder or other spices of your choice

6. Optional: 1-2 Tbsps superfood such as Chia seeds, Flax seeds, Spirulina, Goji berries, etc.

2. One or two handfuls of baby spinach and kale or other greens

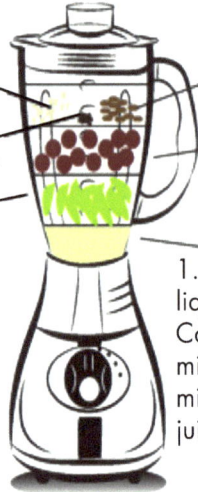

4. Small handfuls of nuts, if you like

3. 1/2 cup to 1 cup of frozen fruit, and/or frozne banana

1. Start off with 1-2 cups of liquid base such as water. Cocout water/Coocunut milk, Almond milk, Soy milk, dairy milk, or fruit juice.

1. **Smoothie liquid base.** The liquid goes into the blender first because it needs to be surrounding the blade in order for the blending process to start properly.
2. **Fruits and vegetables**. The order of these two items doesn't matter that much. I personally like adding vegetables first, then fruits, as the weight of the fruits can push the light vegetables down to be close to the blade.
3. **Special additions.** The additional ingredients, such as protein powder, superfood powders, vitamin powders, nuts or nut butters, and oats, will help balance nutrient content and give your smoothie that extra zing, as well as flavor and thicken the smoothie.
4. **Ice**. If you prefer to use fresh fruit, you may want to add ice cubes to give your smoothie a thicker texture and a cooler temperature. In this cleanse book, we mostly use frozen fruit, so ice is not necessary.
5. Now that you know the order of ingredients that go into the blender, just hit the button and let your blender do its magic.
6. When you see the solid ingredients are all gone and the liquid is fully circulating within the blender, keep

blending for 5–10 seconds. By then, all the contents have been liquefied and are freely circulating. At this point, the liquid at the top should be swirling. Depending on the power of your blender, it may take up to 45 seconds for this to happen.

7. In order for your blender to reach proper circulation, it's important to not put too many ingredients in it. If you have a small personal blender like I do and you can't seem to put everything into the blender at the start, blend the majority of the ingredients first until the liquid is circulating, then add the remaining ingredients.

Bonus Tips

- **Control the thickness.** If you want to thicken your smoothie, add ice. If your smoothie is too thick, add more liquid base.
- **Use frozen ingredients.** The cheapest and most nutritious way to make a smoothie is to use frozen ingredients. Frozen fruits have been harvested and frozen during their peak season to ensure the richest flavor. Normally, ice is not needed if using frozen fruits. Buy your favorite frozen fruits in bulk at a major retailer like Costco—you'll save quite a bit of money.
- **Use bananas.** Bananas are a popular choice in smoothies as they help to thicken the smoothie and provide a neutral taste that goes well with almost everything. We use frozen bananas quite a bit in the cleanse, but if you don't have frozen banana on hand, use a ripe one and add a few cubes of ice.
- **Add superfoods**. Don't waste the precious space in your blender and body. Add plenty of superfoods, which have more than ten times the antioxidant power than most other foods.

SUMMARY

The mental preparation for this cleanse is far more important than the physical preparation. In this chapter you learned to expect and welcome the detox symptoms, prepared to give up your favorite foods for seven days, and found out exactly what to purchase and how to make a perfect smoothie for your cleanse. Next, we will dive into the **actual meals and recipes** for the entire seven days. Are you ready?

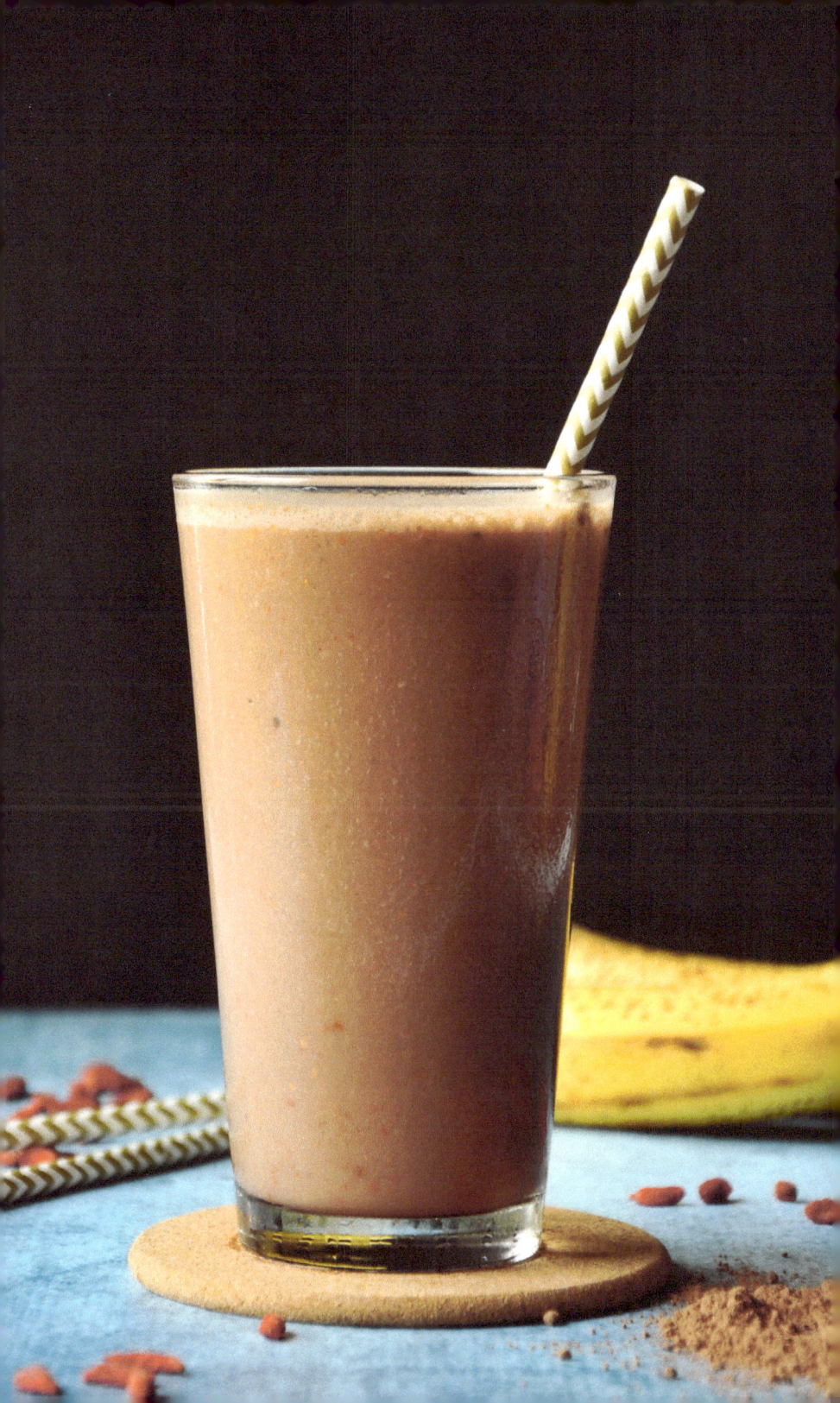

CHAPTER 7

THE MEALS AND RECIPES

All right! You have picked a week and decided to set it as your cleanse week. You have mentally prepared and you believe you can do this. (Yes, you can do it!) You have downloaded the cleanse journal template and printed it out. You have run into the grocery store and grabbed all you need. Let's get started!

In this chapter, there will be a gentle reminder each morning and night to help you stick to the plan.

Some of the smoothies have a non-cleanse version, which is to use fruit juice or coconut water as the full smoothie base. These variations taste better. However, during the cleanse, to prevent blood sugar spike, we tend to use more water and flavor up the smoothies with stevia, which is a natural sweetener contains no calories.

DAY ONE

MORNING REMINDER:

- First thing in the morning: Weigh and measure, then write down the numbers and date on your cleanse journal. Take a photo of your entire body.
- Second thing in the morning: Squeeze half of a lemon into a cup of lukewarm water and drink it up.
- Drink eight cups of water throughout the day.

Breakfast: Goji Green Smoothie

1 frozen banana, cut into chunks
2 cups (handfuls) of spinach and kale, packed
1 tbsp goji berries
¼ cup (1 scoop) vanilla protein powder
1 cup water

Place water, greens, banana, goji berries, and protein powder into a blender. Blend on high speed until ingredients are fully liquefied.

NUTRITION INFORMATION

Serving size: 1   Calories: 365   Calories from Fat: 61   % Daily Value: Total Fat 7g 11%   Saturated fat: 1g 4%   Carbohydrates: 54g 18% Sugar: 17g   Sodium: 226mg 9%   Fiber: 8g 33%   Protein: 29g   Vitamin A 557%   Vitamin C 346%   Calcium 78%   Iron 53%

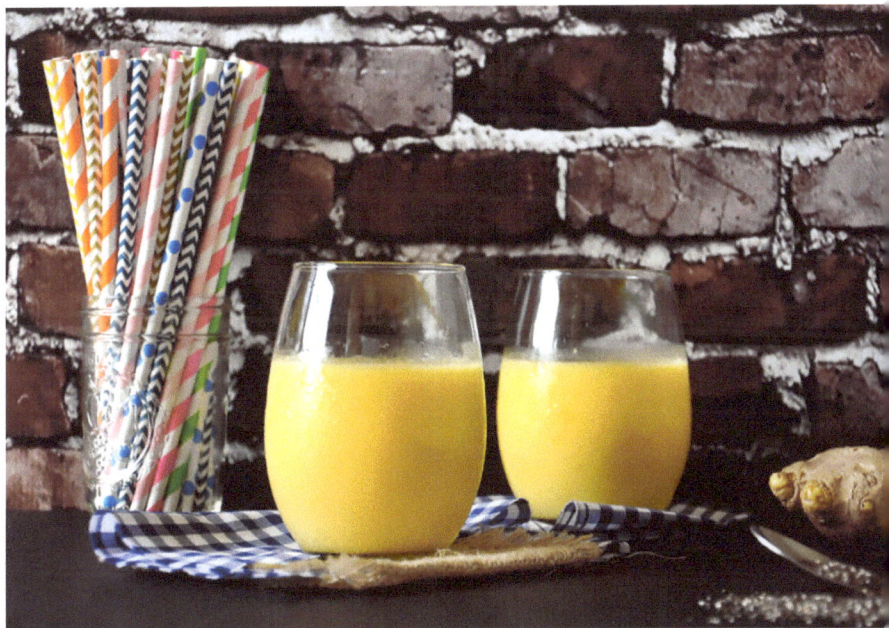

Lunch: Ginger Mango Smoothie

1 cup frozen mango
½ frozen banana, cut into chunks
1-inch chunk ginger
¾ cup water
½ cup orange juice

½ packet stevia
1 tbsp chia seeds (optional)

Place water, orange juice, mango, banana, ginger, stevia, and chia seeds (if using) into your blender, then blend on high speed until all ingredients are fully liquefied.

(*Non-cleanse version of this recipe:* Replace water with orange juice. I personally think there's no need to sweeten it up with stevia if you go full orange juice as the smoothie base.)

NUTRITION INFORMATION

Serving size: 1   Calories: 256   Calories from Fat: 32   % Daily Value: Total Fat 4g 6%   Saturated fat: 1g 3%   Carbohydrates: 56g 19% Sugar: 41g   Sodium: 16mg 1%   Fiber: 8g 31%   Protein: 4g   Vitamin A   41%   Vitamin C 171%   Calcium 10%   Iron 7%

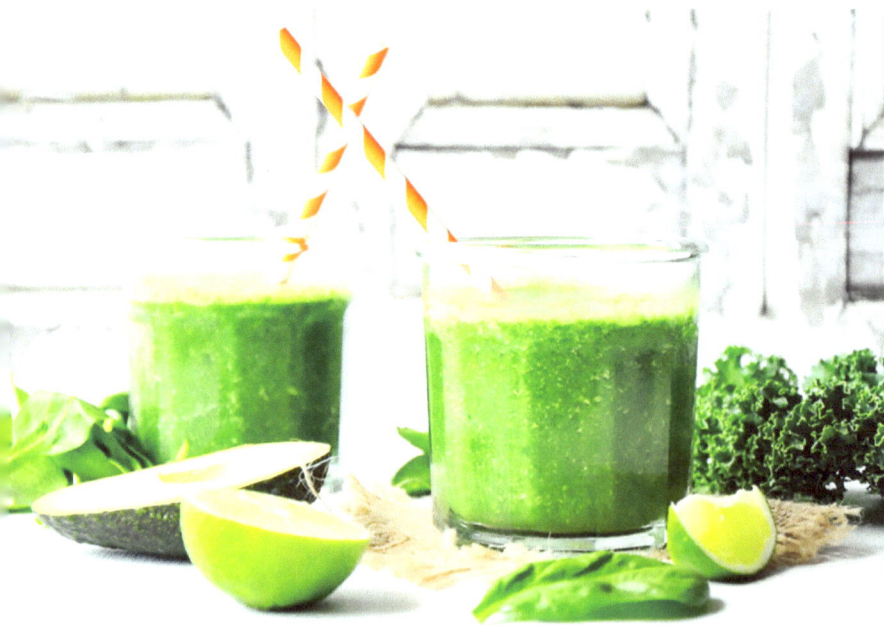

Dinner: Avocado Pineapple Smoothie

½ avocado
1 cup frozen pineapple
½ cup coconut water
¾ cup water
1 cup (handful) of spinach and kale, packed
1 tbsp lime juice
½ packet of stevia
1 tsp spirulina (optional)

Place water, coconut water, and lime juice into your blender, followed by the green leaves. Top with pineapple and avocado, then add stevia and spirulina if using. Blend on high speed until smooth.

(*Non-cleanse version of this recipe:* Replace water with coconut water and omit the stevia.)

NUTRITION INFORMATION

Serving size: 1   Calories: 312   Calories from Fat: 132   % Daily Value: Total Fat 16g 24%   Saturated fat: 2g 12%   Carbohydrates: 44g 15% Sugar: 21g   Sodium: 197mg 8%   Fiber: 12g 50%   Protein: 7g   Vitamin A   267%   Vitamin C 303%   Calcium 19%   Iron 19%

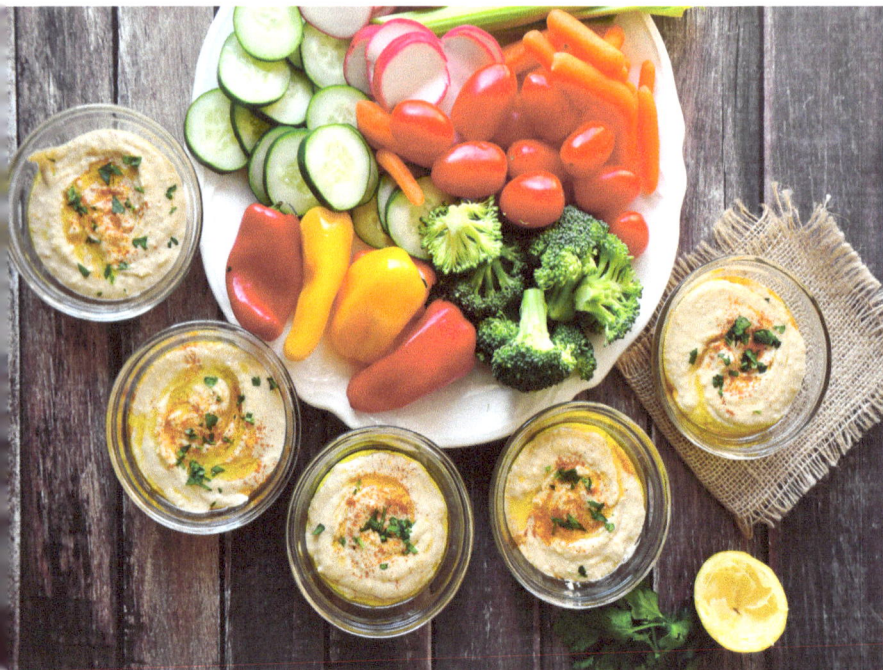

Snack: Classic Hummus

1 (15-oz) can chickpeas, NOT drained
½ cup tahini
2 tbsps extra virgin olive oil
2 tbsps lemon juice
¾ tsp salt
3 cloves garlic
5–10 drops hot sauce (optional)
Chopped fresh parsley and paprika for garnishing

Place all ingredients except parsley and paprika into a food processor. Blend until smooth.

Divide into five portions (½ cup each). Garnish with a little more olive oil, parsley, and paprika. Enjoy with raw, non-starchy vegetables.

You may chop up some fresh veggies like celery, cucumber, and radish. Pack some with you the next day together with one portion of hummus.

NUTRITION INFORMATION

Serving size: 1/5 of recipe   Calories: 238   Calories from Fat: 124   %
Daily Value: Total Fat 15g 23%   Saturated fat: 2g 10%   Carbohy-
drates:22g 7%   Sugar: 1g   Sodium: 527mg 6%   Fiber: 3g 13%
Protein: 9g   Vitamin A 1%   Vitamin C 31%   Calcium 14%   Iron
17%

NIGHT REMINDER:
Before going to bed, document how you felt during the first day
of the cleanse.

DAY TWO

MORNING REMINDER:
- First thing in the morning: Weigh yourself to see if
  you've lost a couple pounds due to your break from
  solid food. Write down the number.
- Second thing in the morning: Drink lemon water.
- Drink eight cups of water throughout the day.

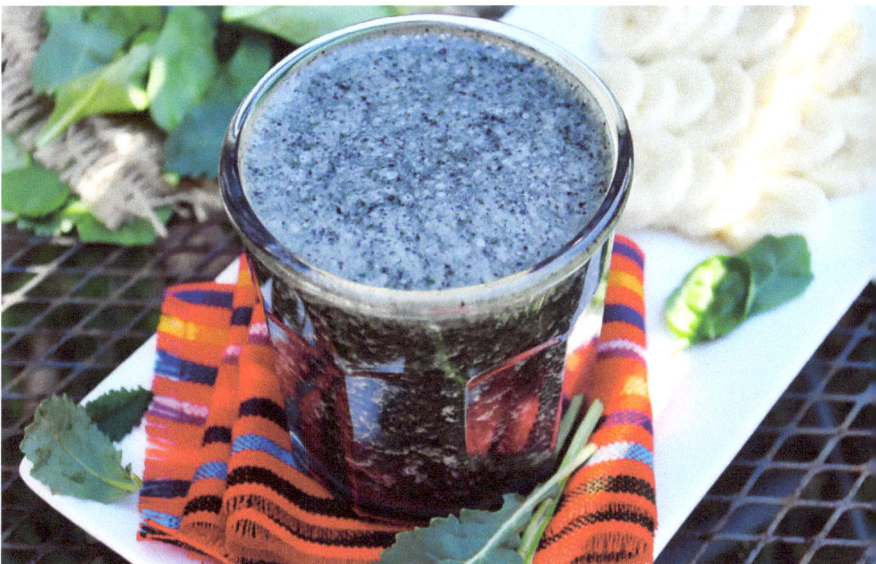

Breakfast and Lunch: Super Power Smoothie

(Double the recipe if you have a big blender that can hold 40 oz. liquid. Otherwise, make the recipe twice in the morning and pack one smoothie for lunch.)

1 cup frozen blueberries
1 cup (handful) kale and spinach, packed
1 ripe banana, broken into chunks
½ cup coconut water
¾ cup water
2 tbsps (½ scoop) vanilla protein powder
½ packet stevia (optional)
1 tsp spirulina (optional)

Place water and coconut water into your blender, then add frozen blueberries followed by green leaves. Top with banana, protein powder, stevia, and spirulina (if using). Blend on high speed until all ingredients are liquefied and smooth.

(*Non-cleanse version of the recipe*: Use 1 ¼ cups coconut water as smoothie base.)

NUTRITION INFORMATION

Serving size: 1   Calories: 299   Calories from Fat: 32   % Daily Value:
Total Fat 4g 6%   Saturated fat: 1g 3%   Carbohydrates: 61g 20%
Sugar: 32g   Sodium: 220mg 9%   Fiber: 11g 43%   Protein: 37g
Vitamin A 274%   Vitamin C 185%   Calcium 32%   Iron 24%

Dinner: Vegetable Salad

5 oz. spring mix
1 cup carrot sticks
Half cucumber, sliced
1 cup red cabbage, sliced
2 cups lettuce, shredded(Feel free to add any other non-starchy raw vegetables like celery, broccoli, and radish.)

7-DAY SUPER SMOOTHIE CLEANSE ACTION PLAN

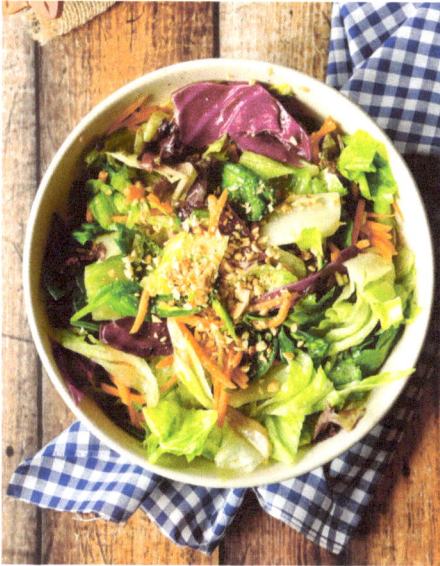

Dressing #1
¼ cup olive oil
2 tbsps lemon juice
1 tbsp Dijon mustard
Salt and pepper to taste

Dressing #2
¼ cup olive oil
1 tbsp lemon juice
1 tbsp Dijon mustard
2 tbsps balsamic vinegar
Salt and pepper to taste

Dressing #3
¼ cup canola oil
¼ cup lime juice
1 tbsp fish sauce
1 tbsp red chili paste
½ tsp siracha
Salt to taste

Dressing #4
¼ cup canola oil
3 tbsps sesame oil
1 ½ tsps minced ginger
2 tbsps cider vinegar
1 tbsp oyster sauce
Black pepper

Pick a dressing. Combine all dressing ingredients in a small bowl. Mix well and set aside. Mix all the fresh vegetables. Pour the dressing over. Stir well and top with two tbsps chopped almonds. Divide it into two portions. Enjoy the first portion for dinner and pack the other for next day's lunch.

NUTRITION INFORMATION

Serving size: 1/2 of recipe   Calories: 1321   Calories from Fat: 1156   % Daily Value: Total Fat 131g 201%   Saturated fat: 73g 9%   Carbohydrates: 42g 14%   Sugar: 14g   Sodium: 1507mg 63%   Fiber: 11g 46%   Protein: 9g   Vitamin A 240%   Vitamin C 254%   Calcium 20%   Iron 21%

NIGHT REMINDER:
Before going to bed, document how you felt during the second day of the cleanse.

DAY THREE

MORNING REMINDER:
- First thing in the morning: Drink lemon water.
- Drink eight cups of water throughout the day.

Breakfast: Avocado Cucumber Smoothie

½ avocado
Juice from 1 lemon
1 ¼ cups water
1 cucumber, cut into chunks
1/3 cup fresh cilantro
¼ cup (1 scoop) vanilla protein powder
1 tbsp ground flaxseed (optional)

Place water and lemon juice into your blender. Add avocado, cilantro, and cucumber. Top with protein powder and flaxseed if using. Blend on high speed until smooth.

(*Non-cleanse version of this*: Replace water with coconut water.)

NUTRITION INFORMATION

Serving size: 1   Calories: 464   Calories from Fat: 213   % Daily Value: Total Fat 25g 39%   Saturated fat: 3g 16%   Carbohydrates: 41g 14%

Sugar: 10g   Sodium: 147mg 6%   Fiber: 15g 59%   Protein: 29g   Vitamin A 62%   Vitamin C 143%   Calcium 66%   Iron 45%

Lunch: Vegetable Salad

Enjoy the salad that you made the night before.

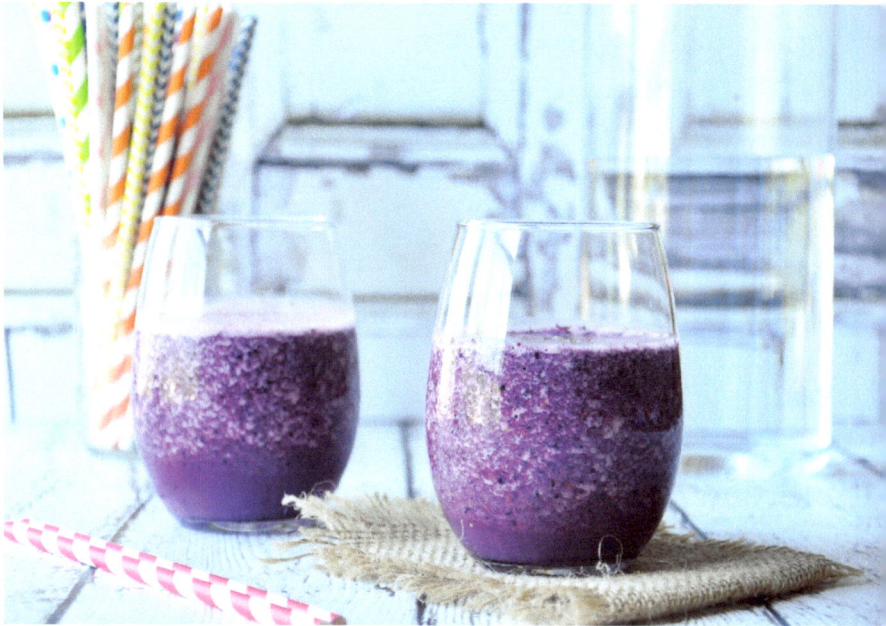

Dinner: Classic Berry Smoothie

1 cup frozen berry mix
1 cup water
¼ cup (1 scoop) vanilla protein powder
¼ cup Greek plain yogurt
1 tbsp chia seeds (optional)
½ packet stevia (optional)

Add water to your blender, followed by frozen berries. Top with yogurt, protein powder, chia seeds, and stevia (if using) and blend on high speed until all ingredients are liquefied and smooth.

(*Non-cleanse version of this recipe*: Replace water with apple juice.)

NUTRITION INFORMATION

Serving size: 1   Calories: 355   Calories from Fat: 90   % Daily Value:
Total Fat 10g 16%   Saturated fat: 2g 10%   Carbohydrates: 37g 12%
Sugar: 15g   Sodium: 154mg 6%   Fiber: 9g 34%   Protein: 27g   Vitamin A 34%   Vitamin C 183%   Calcium 70%   Iron 43%

NIGHT REMINDER:
Before going to bed, document how you felt during the third day of the cleanse.

DAY FOUR

MORNING REMINDER:
- First thing in the morning: Weigh and measure yourself, then write down the numbers and date in your cleanse journal.
- Second thing in the morning: Drink lemon water.
- Drink eight cups of water throughout the day.

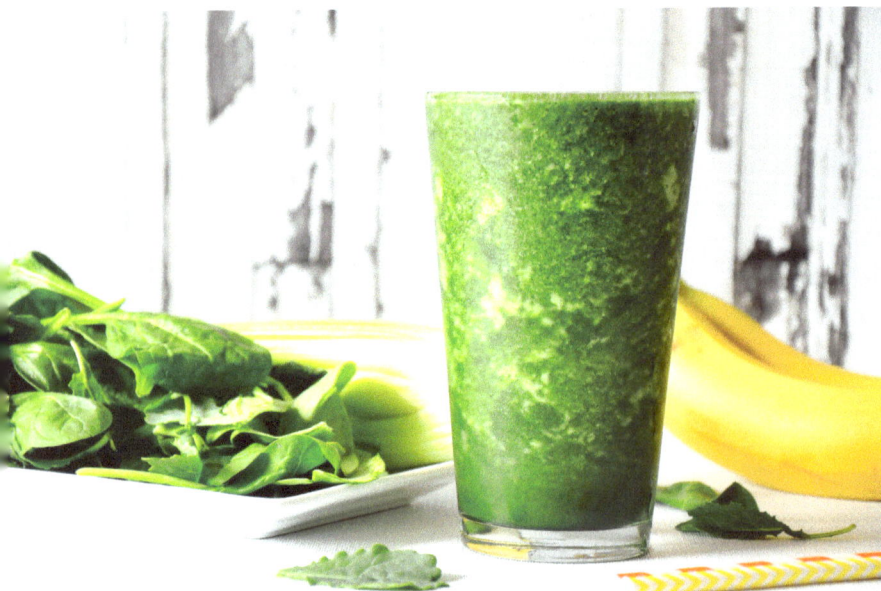

Breakfast and Lunch: Green Lover Smoothie

(Double the recipe if you have a big blender that can hold 40 oz. liquid. Otherwise, make the recipe twice in the morning and pack one smoothie for lunch.)

1 stalk celery, roughly chopped
2 cups (handfuls) spinach and kale, packed
1 frozen banana, cut into chunks
1 cup water
2 tbsps (½ scoop) vanilla protein powder
½ packet stevia
1 tsp spirulina (optional)

Place water in your blender. Add greens and celery, followed by banana. Top with protein powder, stevia, and spirulina (if using). Blend on high speed until smooth.

(*Non-cleanse version of this recipe*: Replace water with coconut water.)

NUTRITION INFORMATION

Serving size: 1   Calories: 244   Calories from Fat: 27   % Daily Value: Total Fat 3g 5%   Saturated fat: 0g 2%   Carbohydrates: 47g 16% Sugar: 16g Sodium: 179mg 7%   Fiber: 8g 32%   Protein: 14g Vitamin A   538%   Vitamin C 324%   Calcium 42%   Iron 32%

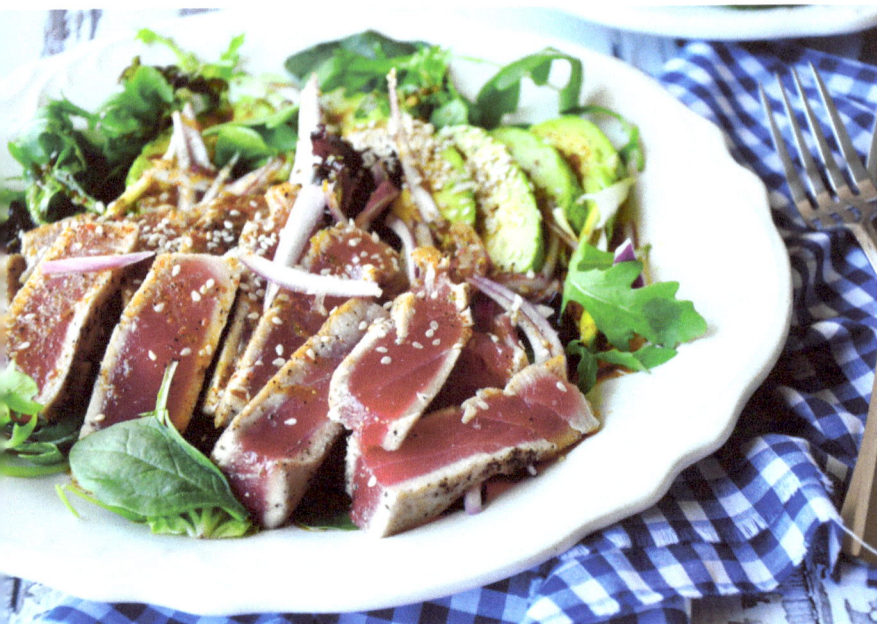

Dinner: Spicy Avocado Seared Tuna Combo

8 oz. tuna steak
1 ripe avocado, sliced
2.5 oz. spring mix (spinach, arugula, cabbage, etc.)
1 small red onion, thinly sliced
2 tbsps white sesame seeds

Dressing:
¼ cup olive oil
Lime zest from half a lime
Juice of 1 lime
½ tsp ground black pepper
1 tbsp soy sauce
½ tsp cayenne pepper

Make the dressing by combining all ingredients in a small bowl. Stir well and divide into two portions.

To sear the tuna, brush some olive oil on each side of the tuna steak. Sprinkle with a dash of salt and pepper. Heat up a sauté pan over high heat for two minutes. Gently place prepared tuna steak into the pan and cook for one minute on each side. Remove from pan and let cool before slicing. Divide into two portions.

On a large plate, arrange one handful of spring mix, half of the sliced onion and half of the sliced avocado together. Place one portion of tuna slices (four oz.) on top and drizzle with one portion of the dressing. Sprinkle with 1 tbsp white sesame seeds and enjoy.

Do the same with the second serving in a container. It's your lunch tomorrow.

NUTRITION INFORMATION

Serving size: 1/2 of recipe   Calories: 638   Calories from Fat: 414   % Daily Value: Total Fat 48g 74%   Saturated fat: 7g 35%   Carbohydrates: 20g 7%   Sugar: 3g   Sodium: 523mg 22%   Fiber: 11g 43%   Protein: 37g   Vitamin A 61%   Vitamin C 52%   Calcium 18% Iron 26%

NIGHT REMINDER:
Before going to bed, document how you felt during the fourth day of the cleanse.

DAY FIVE

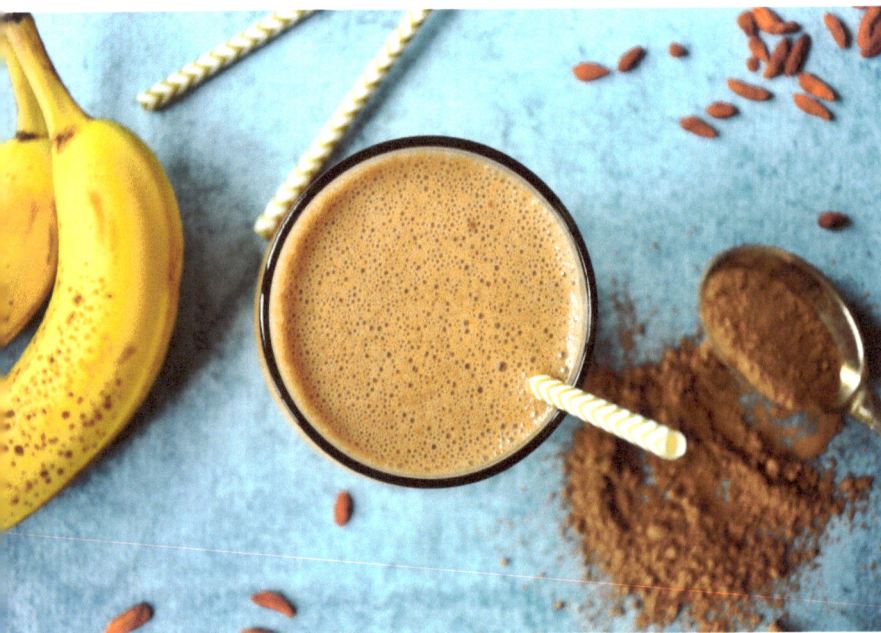

MORNING REMINDER:
- First thing in the morning: Drink lemon water.
- Drink eight cups of water throughout the day.

Breakfast: Chocolate Banana Smoothie

1 cup almond milk/soy milk
1 ½ frozen banana, cut into chunks
1 tbsp cocoa powder
¼ cup Greek plain yogurt
1 tbsp goji berries

Add almond milk/soy milk into your blender, followed by banana. Add yogurt and top with cocoa powder, protein powder, and goji berries. Blend on high speed till smooth.

7-DAY SUPER SMOOTHIE CLEANSE ACTION PLAN

NUTRITION INFORMATION

Serving size: 1   Calories: 317   Calories from Fat: 61   % Daily Value: Total Fat 7g 11%   Saturated fat: 2g 12%   Carbohydrates: 60g 20% Sugar: 34g   Sodium: 145mg 6%   Fiber: 7g 28%   Protein: 11g   Vitamin A   13%   Vitamin C 28%   Calcium 39%   Iron 13%

Lunch: Spicy Avocado Seared Tuna Combo

Enjoy the second serving of the delicious combo you made last night.

Dinner: Kiwi Strawberry Smoothie

½ cup almond milk/soy milk
½ cup water
2 kiwi fruits, peeled
½ cup strawberries
½ frozen banana, cut into chunks
¼ cup Greek plain yogurt
½ packet stevia
1 tbsp ground flaxseed (optional)

Place almond milk and water into your blender. Add kiwi, strawberries, and banana. Top with yogurt, stevia, and flaxseed (if using). Blend on high speed till all ingredients are fully liquefied.

(*Non-cleanse version of this recipe*: Replace water with apple juice and there should be no need to add stevia.)

NUTRITION INFORMATION

Serving size: 1   Calories: 311   Calories from Fat: 80   % Daily Value: Total Fat 9g 14%   Saturated fat: 2g 10%   Carbohydrates: 52g 17% Sugar: 32g   Sodium: 99mg 4%   Fiber: 10g 42%   Protein: 10g   Vitamin A   9%   Vitamin C 304%   Calcium 32%   Iron 11%

NIGHT REMINDER:
Before going to bed, document how you felt during the sixth day of the cleanse.

DAY SIX

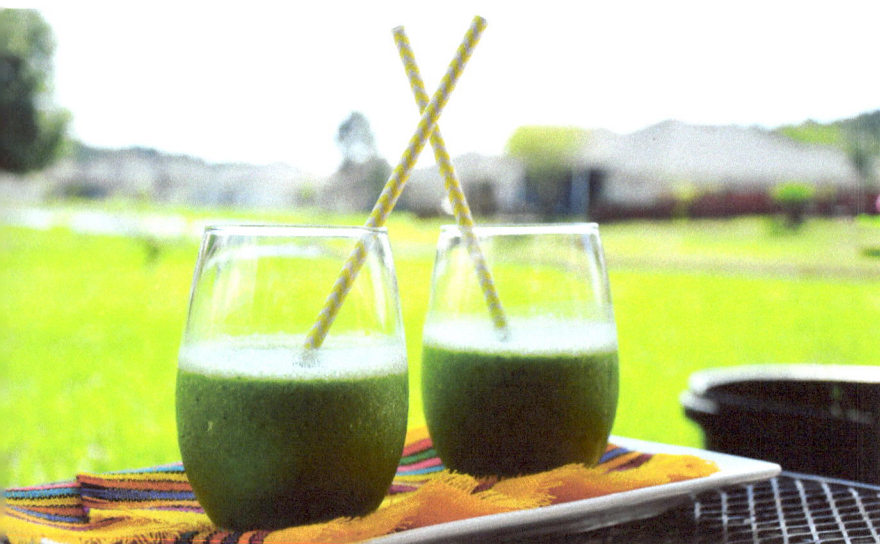

MORNING REMINDER:
- First thing in the morning: Drink lemon water.
- Drink eight cups of water throughout the day.

Breakfast: Peachy Green Smoothie

(Double the recipe if you have a big blender that can hold 40 oz. liquid. Otherwise, make the recipe twice in the morning and pack one smoothie for lunch.)

1 cup almond milk/soy milk
½ cup frozen peaches
½ frozen banana, cut into chunks
1 cup (handful) spinach and kale, packed
2 tbsps (½ scoop) vanilla protein powder
2 tbsps ground flaxseed (optional)

Place almond milk/soy milk into your blender. Add greens and peaches, followed by protein powder and flaxseed (if using).

Blend on high speed until smooth.

NUTRITION INFORMATION

Serving size: 1   Calories: 364   Calories from Fat: 54   % Daily Value: Total Fat 6g 9%   Saturated fat: 1g 4%   Carbohydrates: 66g 22%   Sugar: 44g   Sodium: 206mg 9%   Fiber: 7g 26%   Protein: 17g   Vitamin A 288%   Vitamin C 362%   Calcium 58%   Iron 28%

Dinner: Healthy Quinoa Bowl

½ cup quinoa
1 cup broccoli florets, finely chopped
5 oz. mixed vegetables (carrots, peas, green beans)
¼ cup red onion, diced
1 cup red bell pepper, diced
1 stem green onion, finely chopped
1 tbsp cilantro leaves, chopped
1 tsp dried basil

For the dressing:
2 tbsps fresh lemon juice
1 tbsp Dijon mustard
2 tbsps olive oil
¾ tsp sea salt
¼ tsp ground black pepper

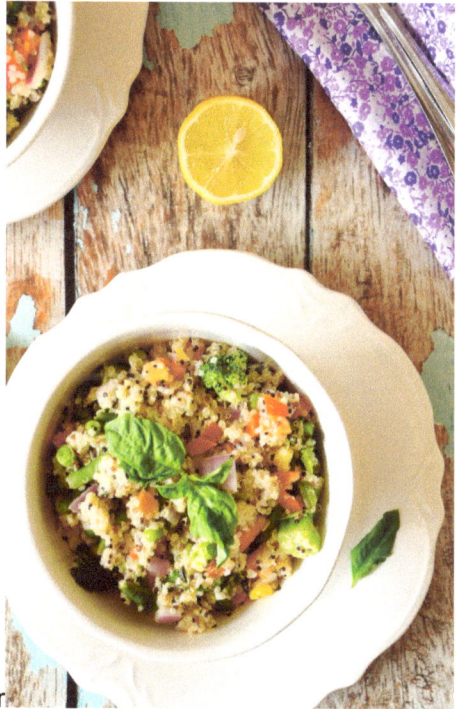

Rinse quinoa under cold water and drain. Place it into a pot and cover with one cup water. Bring to a boil, then turn down the heat, cover, and simmer for 12–14 minutes, or until all of the water is absorbed. Remove from the heat and keep covered for five more minutes. Remove from heat and fluff it with a fork; let cool.

In a saucepan, bring two cups water to a boil. Place mixed vegetables and chopped broccoli into the saucepan (make sure vegetables are covered by water). Cook over medium-high heat for five to six minutes. Stir occasionally. Drain and set aside.

In a small bowl, combine lemon juice, Dijon mustard, olive oil, sea salt, basil, and ground black pepper. Mix well.

In a large bowl, combine cooked vegetables, red onion, bell pepper, cilantro, and green onion. Add quinoa and pour the dressing over. Stir until even. Divide it in half. Enjoy half for dinner and pack the other half for next day's lunch.

NUTRITION INFORMATION

Serving size: 1/2 of recipe   Calories: 280   Calories from Fat: 38   %
Daily Value: Total Fat 4g 7%   Saturated fat: 1g 3%   Carbohydrates:
54g 18%   Sugar: 6g   Sodium: 1025mg 43%   Fiber: 11g 44%
Protein: 12g   Vitamin A 144%   Vitamin C 306%   Calcium 12%
Iron 26%

NIGHT REMINDER:
Before going to bed, document how you felt during the sixth day of the cleanse.

DAY SEVEN

MORNING REMINDER:
- First thing in the morning: Drink lemon water.
- Drink eight cups of water throughout the day.

Breakfast: Crazy Berry Smoothie

¾ cup almond milk/soy milk
½ cup water
1 cup frozen mixed berries
½ ripe banana
¼ cup (1 scoop) vanilla protein powder
1 tsp chia seeds (optional)

Place water and almond milk/soy milk into your blender, followed by mixed berries and banana. Add protein powder and chia seeds (if using). Blend on high speed till all ingredients are fully liquefied.

NUTRITION INFORMATION

Serving size: 1   Calories: 397   Calories from Fat: 83   % Daily Value:
Total Fat 9g 14%   Saturated fat: 1g 5%   Carbohydrates: 54g 18%
Sugar: 26g   Sodium: 206mg 9%   Fiber: 8g 34%   Protein: 29g   Vitamin A 40%   Vitamin C 191%   Calcium 81%   Iron 45%

Lunch: Healthy Quinoa Bowl

Enjoy the quinoa bowl you made last night.

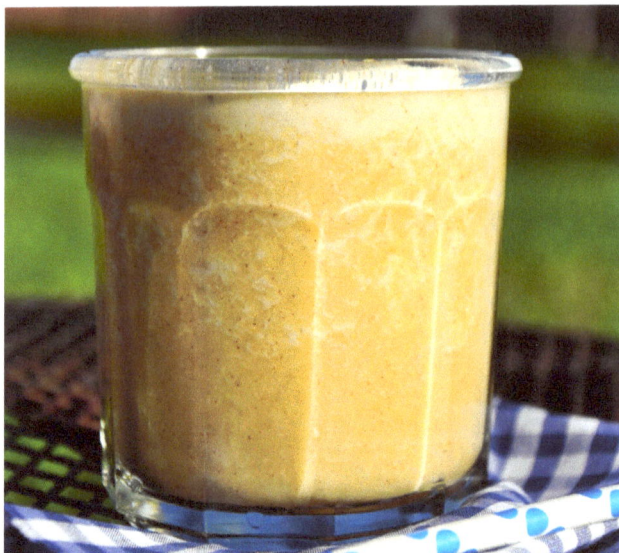

Dinner: Cinnamon Peach Dance

1 cup water
½ cup almond milk/soy milk
1 cup frozen peach
1-inch chunk ginger
½ tsp ground cinnamon
¼ cup (1 scoop) vanilla protein powder
1 tbsp ground flaxseed (optional)

Add water and almond milk/soy milk into your blender. Place peach and ginger in, then add cinnamon, protein powder, and flaxseed (if using). Blend until smooth.

(*Non-cleanse version of this recipe*: Replace water with orange juice.)

NUTRITION INFORMATION

Serving size: 1   Calories: 521   Calories from Fat: 104   % Daily Value: Total Fat 12g 18%   Saturated fat: 1g 6%   Carbohydrates: 80g 27% Sugar: 62g   Sodium: 195mg 8%   Fiber: 9g 37%   Protein: 29g   Vitamin A 50%   Vitamin C 423%   Calcium 73%   Iron 41%

NIGHT REMINDER:
Before going to bed, document how you felt during the seventh day of the cleanse.

DAY EIGHT

MORNING REMINDER:
- First thing in the morning: Weigh and measure yourself to see your final results. You might want to take a photo of your entire body again to compare with the photo that you took seven days ago.
- Second thing in the morning: Continue drinking lemon water...

CONGRATULATIONS! You have successfully finished the Seven-Day Super Smoothie Cleanse Action Plan!

SUMMARY

You have just gone through the entire meal plan and action plan of this seven-day cleanse. Although it's convenient to stick with the designed recipes, remember that the plan is customizable. Check out the appendix of this book for more smoothie and solid food combo recipes. Just be sure to follow the cleanse agenda in chapter 4.

So, the cleanse is over. But your healthy lifestyle is just getting started!

Wondering what to do to maintain the amazing results you got from the cleanse? Want to continue losing one or two pounds every week, even after the cleanse? In the next chapter, I will show you how to do that. Read on.

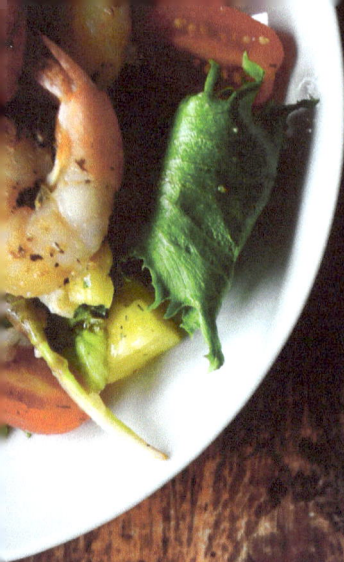

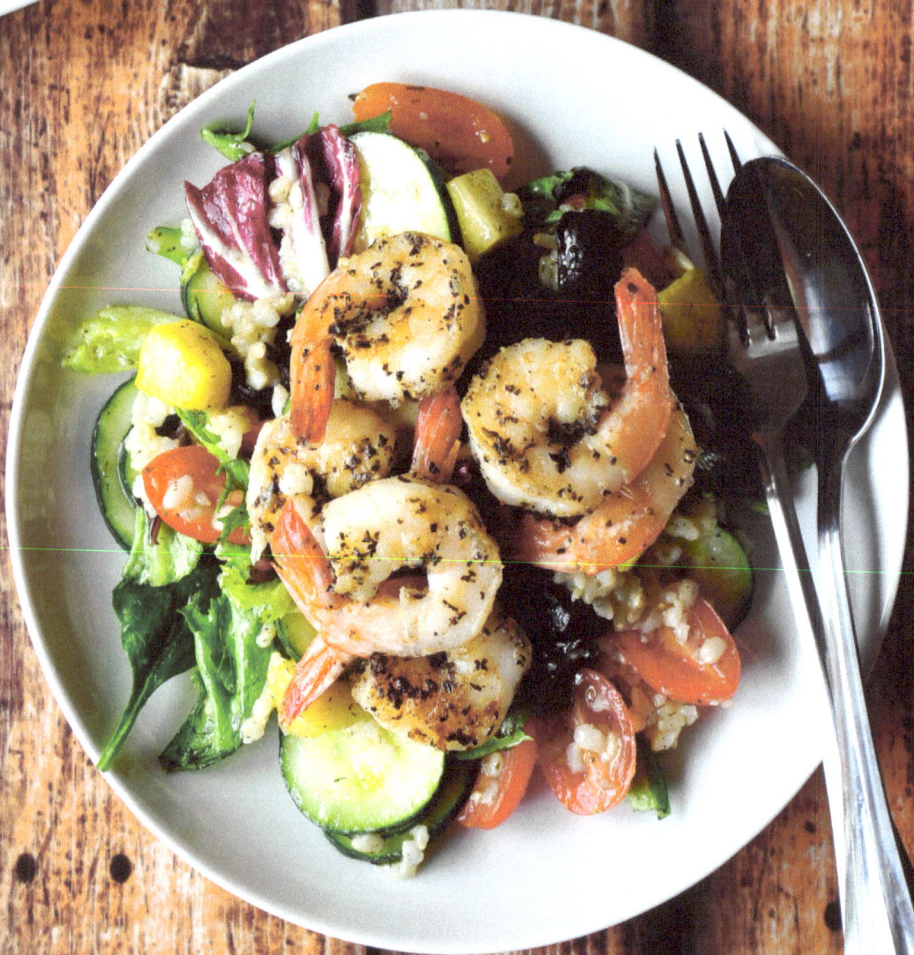

CHAPTER 8

WHAT TO DO AFTER THE CLEANSE

Congratulations!!

You have finished your seven-day cleanse and successfully detox-ified your body! Great job!

Whether you have lost a few pounds, dropped a couple pant sizes, or simply felt better than before, your body system has obtained a complete reboot as needed.

The question is, "Now what?"

If you're like I was, on the first day of the cleanse, you told your-self that you would have a large bowl of pho, a Five Guy burger, BBQ ribs, steak, cheesecake, lots of cheese, coffee, wine, and all your other favorite food after seven days.

Now that it's over, you can finally eat whatever you want again. But you are hesitating, because you want to keep what you have worked so hard for over the past seven days. You are afraid that you are going to lose the results quickly if you just let it go and start eating fried chicken.

It's good that you hesitated. Your concern is totally legitimate.

Weight loss can happen in a week, or even overnight through a detoxification. But it's very easy to gain those pounds back if you don't do anything to maintain. Losing one to two pounds every week is considered healthy. This plan helps place you at a good starting point.

Now let's talk about the maintenance. Don't worry, I won't throw a NO Food List in your face this time. On the contrary, you really don't have to give up what you love. This chapter is about changing your eating habits and introducing you to a new lifestyle.

BALANCE YOUR MEALS

Drink Lemon Water Every Morning

Keep drinking lemon water first thing in the morning on an empty stomach, every day. This is something I would strongly recommend you do in the long run. When we wake up in the morning, our body tissues are dehydrated from the previous night and are in need of water to push out toxins and rejuvenate the cells. Adding lemon to water not only quenches thirst better than any other beverage, but also nourishes our bodies with vitamins, minerals, and trace elements. In other words, lemon with water can be considered the best natural energy booster available. Below are some of the major benefits that drinking lemon water every morning can bring:

1. Hydrates your body
2. Improves digestion
3. Boosts energy
4. Weight loss aid
5. Antibacterial and antiviral properties
6. Boosts brain power
7. Boosts immune system
8. Promotes healthy and rejuvenated skin
9. Alkalizes your body
10. Reduces mucus and phlegm
11. Anti-cancer properties
12. Reduces inflammation
13. Cleansing properties
14. Freshens breath
15. Reduces caffeine craving

Drink a Super Smoothie Every Day

We've discussed a few benefits of drinking super smoothies in chapter 3. Let's see why you should develop the habit of making and drinking super smoothies on a daily basis:

1. Drink your daily vegetables and fruits. With smoothies, you don't have to eat your vegetables and fruits — you can simply drink them to ensure your body's daily nutritional needs.
2. Smoothies can be any meal of the day. You have had smoothies for breakfast, lunch, and dinner during the cleanse, so you know how flexible a smoothie can be — not to mention that you can take it to go if you need to.
3. Quick and easy. Smoothies take no time to prepare compared to other meals.
4. Detox, easier weight loss, and improved digestion. That's what this book is about. :)
5. Energy boost to both your body and your brain. Supply your body and brain with the right fuel of nutrients in the short and long term. Improve your focus and mental clarity.
6. Build lean muscle. Add protein powder to your already nutrient-rich smoothie post-workout. This helps with muscle recovery and rebuilding.
7. The best way to consume superfood supplements. Add chia seeds, flaxseed, spirulina, maca root powder, goji berries, etc. to your smoothies to supply your body with extra nutrients that are not usually contained in our normal meals.
8. Improve sleep quality. It's almost guaranteed that you'll have deeper sleep if you consume super smoothies on a regular basis. You've probably already experienced this with the cleanse.
9. Delicious. Healthy eating as tasty as it gets. With so many super smoothie recipes in this book, as well as on the internet, finding your favorites or even coming up with your own is a breeze.
10. Beauty. Don't you want radiant skin, hair, and nails? The variety of vitamins and minerals in super smoothies provides exactly what your body needs to make your skin and hair glow.

I could go on with this list, but you are well aware that drinking a super smoothie every day is a great investment for better health in the long haul.

Shift Your Daily Food Focus

Work and life balance is important to productivity. Similarly, meal balance is crucial to weight loss. Balance your intake of protein, carbs, fat, and dairy every day. Try to eat a bit of everything, not just one or two things. And, of course, make your meals delicious!

Before you go back to whole foods, try to shift your daily food focus to the following list of foods for as long as possible.

Healthy whole grains: Quinoa, brown rice, 100% whole-grain or whole wheat pasta, 100% whole-grain cereal, millet, oats.

Seafood: Salmon, tuna, sardines, herring, lake trout, clams, shrimp, oysters, scallops.

Meat: Lean beef such as flank, sirloin, round steak, filets, or extra-lean ground beef; lean pork such as tenderloin and loin chops. (Focus on the cuts of meat with little or no marbling.)

Skinless poultry: Turkey and chicken.

Beans and legumes: Black beans, kidney beans, navy beans, pinto beans, white beans, lentils, split yellow and green beans.

Dairy: Reasonable amounts of cheese and yogurt.

Nuts: Almonds, cashews, walnuts, sunflower seeds, pumpkin seeds, sesame seeds, chia seeds, hemp seeds, tahini (choose raw, unsalted nuts).

Oils: Olive oil, canola oil, coconut oil, and avocado oil.

Whether you cook at home or eat out, try to choose the foods listed above as much as possible after the cleanse. They will help you continue to lose weight and stay healthy.

If you struggle with cooking, your **free bonus** *Post Cleanse Meals* is exactly what you need to make delicious meals that can help maintain your results and continue losing weight after a cleanse. All recipes in this free recipe book are made with the recommended ingredients above. Preparation time is no more than 15 minutes. Download your free copy at
http://gourmetpersuasian.com/cleansebonus

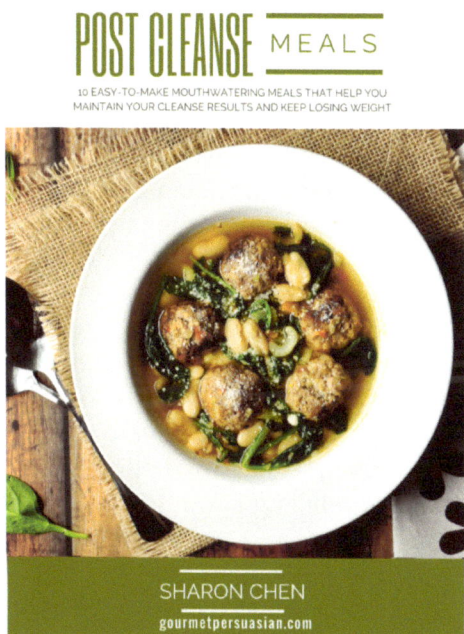

EXERCISE

You lost a few pounds over the past seven days, and you don't want to gain those pounds back again. Instead, you want to lose more, right? Exercise can help you prevent excess weight gain and help maintain weight loss. The more intense the activity, the more calories you burn.

Weight control is just one of the many benefits that regular exercise and physical activity can provide. Other benefits include better sleep, disease prevention, and energy boosts, as well as improved mood.

Regardless of your age, sex, and physically ability, the benefits of exercise are yours for the taking. During the cleanse, I recommend exercising gently and resting more. After the cleanse, regular exercise for at least 30 minutes per day is very much encouraged.

Exercise can be fun. If you don't like running on a treadmill, you don't have to. Pick the activities that you like and that suit you instead of doing what everyone else is doing. Enjoy the outdoors or simply engage in activities that make you happy. Physical activity can also help you connect with family or friends in a fun social setting. So, go to a rock climbing gym, take a dance class, hit the hiking trails, or join a soccer team. If you get bored, try something new.

For example, I was quite a fast runner and used to enjoy marathons. However, after going through an arthroscopic knee surgery on each of my knees, with rivets being implanted seven years ago, I permanently said goodbye to running. Instead, I started doing exercise that has low impact on my knees, like swimming. I find that swimming unwinds my mind when my body moves in the same rhythm.

If you can't do an actual workout, get more active throughout the day in simple ways—by taking the stairs instead of the elevator, walking instead of driving if it's a short distance, or biking to your favorite coffee shop a few blocks away.

Outdoor activities might not always be your jam. This may be because of bad weather, or simply because you want to stay in for the day. Guess what? You still have plenty of options for exercising at home. Here is a list of free exercise programs I personally use to help me stay fit. I hope you find them helpful:

- Less intense (for women): **Full-body workout** (http://bit.ly/14vgUfU), **arm workout** (http://bit.ly/1lvmPRJ), **leg workout** (http://bit.ly/1EEGcrg), **runway core** (http://bit.ly/1B6olK0), and **runway butt** (http://bit.ly/1QM2pGf) are all part of the Train Like an Angel Series conducted by Victoria's Secret models. Each workout takes about 15–20 minutes to complete. Enjoy music videos or TV shows during the workouts once you memorize all the steps in each routine. Trust me, they are pretty easy to remember. There are a lot more workouts in the Train Like an Angel series, which you can find for free on YouTube. The five workouts listed above are my favorites, and have been treating my body very well.

- Intense: **7-Minute Workout** (http://7-min.com/) is a highly effective program that can be done at home or in a hotel room. Each of the 12 exercises scientifically designed into the program take 25 seconds to finish, and you get 10 seconds rest between them. All you need is your body weight, a wall, a chair, and seven minutes!

- Very intense: **FreeLetics** (http://freeletics.com/en) includes high intensity workouts, personalized coaching, and total freedom workouts that you can do anywhere using your body weight only.

In a nutshell, developing healthy eating habits combined with an exercise routine that works for you is going to help you control weight and stay healthy after the cleanse. After all, we should enjoy the life that we deserve—eating delicious food, doing meaningful work, being happy, and staying healthy. It all starts with the new lifestyle that you are about to experience. Take action and get results, my friend!

CONCLUSION

Thank you so, so much for taking the time to read this book If you've decided to try the Seven-Day Super Smoothie Cleanse Action Plan, I want to let you know that I really appreciate your courage and commitment in taking the challenge, improving your health, and changing your eating habits for a healthier lifestyle!

If you've had trouble losing weight for a long time, the cleanse plan in this book can place you in a good position to start shedding pounds. Nothing is impossible. The hardest part is getting started.

If you get a relatively high score from the detox quiz, take the quiz again one to two weeks after you complete the cleanse. You will get a different result.

If you are a super healthy person who doesn't need to lose weight or has a toxin-free body, I hope you enjoy the delicious recipes included in the cleanse. I also hope that the information in this book is useful, and that you will share it with the people you know who need a little push to become aware of how important it is to eliminate toxins from our bodies once in a while.

If you have enjoyed reading this book, or you have achieved amazing results from the cleanse plan, please kindly **leave a review on Amazon**. By sharing your cleanse experience with others, you are helping more people to learn about detoxification and encouraging them to live healthier lives. Furthermore, your feedback is extremely important to me, as it will help me create more healthy eating plans, recipes, and books for you to enjoy.

Lastly, please share this book with your friends and families that you think will benefit from the cleans. I am looking forward to hearing your success stories, and theirs!

APPENDIX

MORE SMOOTHIE AND COMBO RECIPES FOR YOUR CLEANSE

SMOOTHIES

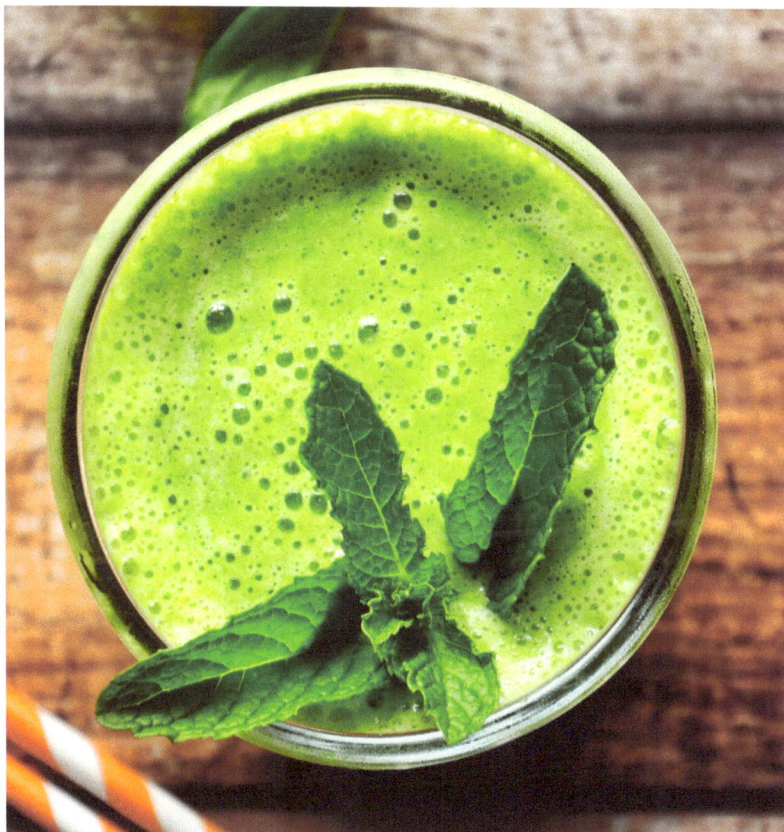

Minty Pineapple Green Smoothie

½ cup coconut water
½ cup water
1 cup frozen pineapple
1 cup (handful) kale and spinach, packed
6 mint leaves

¼ cup Greek plain yogurt
½ packet Stevia (optional)
2 tbsps ground flaxseed (optional)

Add coconut water and water into your blender, followed by green leaves and mint. Add yogurt, then pineapple. Top with stevia and flaxseed (if using) and blend on high speed until all ingredients are fully liquefied.

(*Non-cleanse version of this recipe*: Use 1 cup coconut water as the smoothie base.)

NUTRITION INFORMATION

Serving size: 1   Calories: 185   Calories from Fat: 26   % Daily Value: Total Fat 3g 5%   Saturated fat: 2g 8%   Carbohydrates: 37g 12% Sugar: 23g   Sodium: 213mg 9%   Fiber: 6g 23%   Protein: 7g   Vitamin A   266%   Vitamin C 285%   Calcium 25%   Iron 16%

Tropical Fruit Smoothie

½ cup coconut water
¾ cup water
1 ripe banana
½ cup frozen pineapple
½ cup frozen mango
¼ cup Greek plain yogurt
½ packet stevia
2 tbsps ground flaxseed (optional)

Place coconut water and water into your blender. Add pineapple and mango, followed by yogurt and banana. Top with stevia and blend on high speed until smooth.

(*Non cleanse version*: Replace water and stevia with coconut water.)

NUTRITION INFORMATION

Serving size: 1   Calories: 258   Calories from Fat: 26   % Daily Value: Total Fat 3g 5%   Saturated fat: 2g 9%   Carbohydrates: 58g 19% Sugar: 40g   Sodium: 164mg 7%   Fiber: 7g 27%   Protein: 5g   Vitamin A 22%   Vitamin C 138%   Calcium 13%   Iron 6%

Cherry-Berry Smoothie

½ cup almond milk/soy milk
¾ cup water
½ cup frozen cherries
½ cup strawberries
¼ cup Greek plain yogurt
¼ cup (1 scoop) vanilla protein powder
½ packet stevia (optional)
1 tbsp chia seeds (optional)

Place almond milk/soy milk and water into your blender, then add cherries, strawberries, and yogurt, followed by protein powder and chia seeds (if using). Blend on high speed until smooth.

(*Non-cleanse version of this recipe*: Use almond milk/soy milk as the full smoothie base.)

NUTRITION INFORMATION

Serving size: 1   Calories: 451   Calories from Fat: 108   % Daily Value: Total Fat 12g 19%   Saturated fat: 2g 12%   Carbohydrates: 58g 19% Sugar: 40g   Sodium: 206mg 9%   Fiber: 9g 34%   Protein: 31g   Vitamin A 42%   Vitamin C 115%   Calcium 84%   Iron 41%

Cilantro Mango Smoothie

1 cup water
½ frozen banana
1 cup frozen mango
1 cup fresh cilantro
1 cup (handful) spinach and kale, packed
¼ cup (1 scoop) vanilla protein powder
1 tsp spirulina (optional)

Add water to your blender, followed by cilantro, spinach, and kale. Then add mango and banana. Push it down if your blender is a small personal one. Top with protein powder and spirulina (if using). Blend on high speed until ingredients are fully liquefied.

(*Non-cleanse version of this recipe:* Replace water with coconut water.)

NUTRITION INFORMATION

Serving size: 1   Calories: 370   Calories from Fat: 60   % Daily Value: Total Fat 7g   10%   Saturated fat: 1g 4%   Carbohydrates: 56g 19% Sugar: 32g   Sodium: 182mg 8%   Fiber: 8g 30%   Protein: 27g   Vitamin A   351%   Vitamin C 295%   Calcium 69%   Iron   44%

Almond Butter Banana Smoothie

1 cup almond milk
1 ripe banana
2 tbsps almond butter
¼ cup (1 scoop) vanilla protein powder
2 tbsps ground flaxseed (optional)
5 ice cubes

Place almond milk into your blender. Add banana, almond butter, and ice. Top with protein powder and ground flaxseed (if using). Blend on high speed until smooth.

NUTRITION INFORMATION

Serving size: 1 Calories: 309   Calories from Fat: 51   % Daily Value: Total Fat 8g   13%   Saturated fat: 1g 3%   Carbohydrates: 37g 12% Sugar: 16g   Sodium: 159mg 7%   Fiber: 4g 18%   Protein: 24g   Vitamin A 32%   Vitamin C 48%   Calcium 102%   Iron 33%

COMBOS

Asian Pan-Fried Scallop Quinoa Combo

8 oz. bay scallops, thawed
1 cup cherry tomatoes, halved
½ cup uncooked quinoa
1 (5-oz.) package spring mix
3 tbsps teriyaki marinade/sauce

Asian Ginger Sauce:
1 tbsp ginger, minced
1 tbsp oyster sauce
1 tbsp soy sauce
2 tsps sesame oil

Cook quinoa in a rice cooker just like you cook regular rice. If you don't have a rice cooker, rinse quinoa under cold water and drain. Place it into a saucepan and cover with 1 cup water. Bring to a boil, then turn down the heat, cover, and simmer for 12 to 14 minutes, or until all of the water is absorbed. Remove from the heat and keep covered for five more minutes. Uncover and let cool.

Combine all the ginger sauce ingredients in a small bowl. Mix well and set aside.

Add tomatoes and spring mix into the saucepan with the cooked quinoa. Pour sauce over and stir until even. Transfer half of the quinoa mix to a serving plate.

Heat up a sauté pan over high heat for two minutes. Add teriyaki sauce into the pan, followed by the scallops. Switch heat to medium-high. Cook for two minutes without stirring. Let the flavor sear in. Stir, then cook for another one to two minutes until scallops are done. Top the quinoa mix with half of the scallops and enjoy!

Pack the other half of the quinoa mix and the rest of scallops for the next day's lunch. When ready to serve, warm up the scallops and place on top of the quinoa mix.

NUTRITION INFORMATION

Serving size: 1/2 of recipe Calories: 393   Calories from Fat: 151   % Daily Value: Total Fat 17g 26%   Saturated fat: 2g 12%   Carbohydrates: 39g 13%   Sugar: 3g   Sodium: 1167mg 49%   Fiber: 5g 21%   Protein: 22g   Vitamin A 120%   Vitamin C 32%   Calcium 7%   Iron 19%

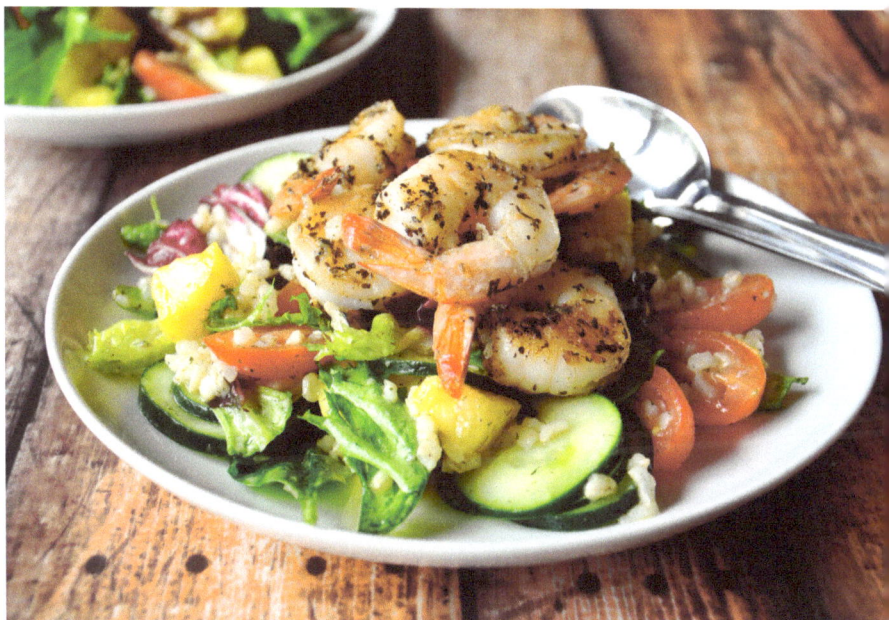

Grilled Shrimp Brown Rice Combo

8 oz. jumbo shrimp (about 12 to 14 shrimp), peeled, deveined, tail-on
1 cup cooked brown rice
1 cup cherry tomatoes, halved
1 medium cucumber, sliced
1 cup fresh pineapple, diced
2.5 oz. spring mix

Shrimp seasoning:
1 tbsp olive oil
¼ tsp sea salt
¼ tsp ground black pepper
½ tsp garlic powder
½ tsp dried basil

Combo dressing:
1 tsp dried dill
1 clove garlic, minced
2 tbsps olive oil
1 tbsp fresh lemon juice
Salt and pepper to taste (¼ tsp for each worked perfectly for me)

Prepare or thaw the shrimp (if using frozen shrimp). Pat dry with a paper towel. In a medium bowl, combine shrimp with shrimp seasonings. Prepare grill and grill two minutes on each side or until shrimps are done.

In a large mixing bowl, combine brown rice, pineapple, spring mix, cherry tomatoes, and cucumber. Mix combo dressing in a small bowl and pour over combo ingredients. Toss to mix well. Divide brown rice mix into two portions. Place six shrimp on the first portion and enjoy!

Pack the rest of the brown rice mix and shrimp for the next day's lunch.

NUTRITION INFORMATION

Serving size: 1/2 of recipe   Calories: 404   Calories from Fat: 92   %
Daily Value: Total Fat 10g 16%   Saturated fat: 2g 9%   Carbohydrates:
48g 16%   Sugar: 14g   Sodium: 1469mg 61%   Fiber: 6g 24%
Protein: 31g   Vitamin A 79%   Vitamin C 103%   Calcium 20%
Iron 16%

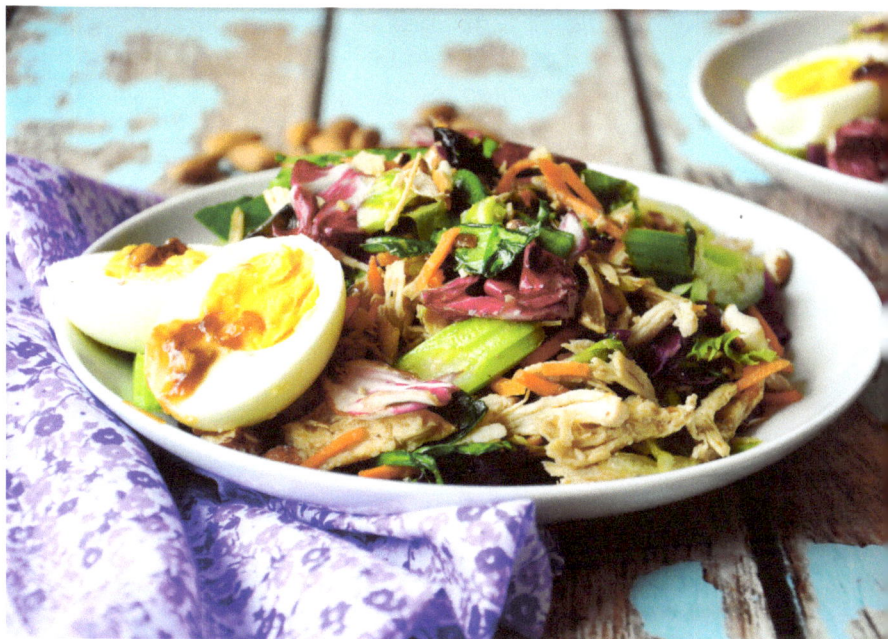

Rainbow Chicken Combo

2 cups cooked and shredded chicken
2.5 oz. spring mix
2 hard-boiled eggs, halved
1 cup red cabbage, shredded
1 cup celery, shredded
1 cup carrot matchsticks
1 stalk green onion, chopped
2 cups Romaine lettuce, shredded
Sliced almonds and white sesame seeds for topping

Combo dressing ingredients:
2 tbsps oyster sauce
1 tbsp Thai red chili paste
1 tbsp sesame oil
1 tbsp grated ginger
Freshly ground black pepper

Combine dressing ingredients in a small bowl and set aside.

Place chicken and all vegetables into a large mixing bowl. Pour dressing over and mix well. Sprinkle with freshly ground black pepper. Garnish with chopped almond and white sesame seeds.

Divide chicken combo into two portions. Add one hard-boiled egg to each portion. Enjoy one portion for dinner and pack the other for the next day's lunch.

NUTRITION INFORMATION

Serving size: 1/2 of recipe   Calories: 471   Calories from Fat: 179   %
Daily Value: Total Fat 20g 31%   Saturated fat: 5g 23%   Carbohydrates: 18g 6%   Sugar: 7g   Sodium: 273mg 11%   Fiber: 6g 25%
Protein: 54g   Vitamin A 341%   Vitamin C 80%   Calcium 19%
Iron 27%

YOUR FREE BONUS

Post Cleanse Meals: 10 Easy-To-Make Mouthwatering Meals That Help You Maintain Your Cleanse Results and Keep Losing Weight

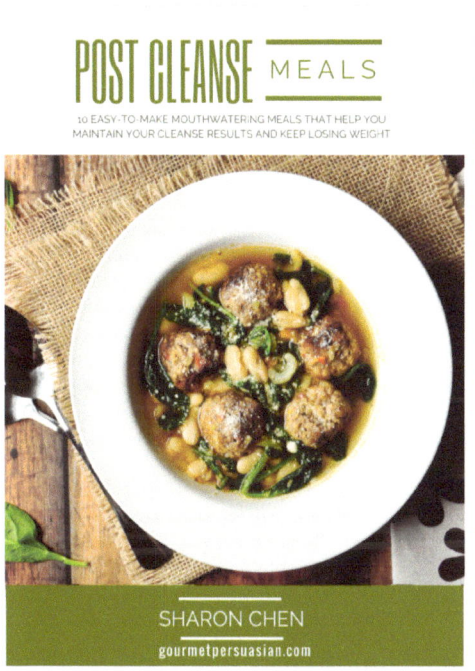

http://gourmetpersuasian.com/cleansebonus

ABOUT THE AUTHOR

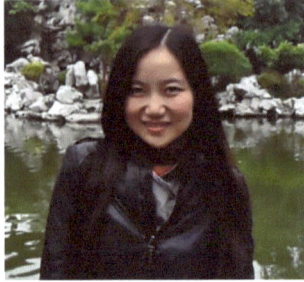

Hi there! I am Sharon, a former real estate professional who turned to be a healthy food blogger at GourmePersuasian.Com.

When I was growing up, my mom had a tremendous influence on me through her passion for cooking, and how important cooking and eating at home were to a vibrant family life. It was not until I moved away from my hometown of Shanghai, China to the States with my husband that I realized what cooking really means.

It's a way of presenting and sharing love by turning a wide range of fresh ingredients into a plate of delicious and beautiful looking food to nurture those who I care about. It's a way of giving thanks.

That's why I strive to encourage more people to cook whole foods at home in a simple and healthy way by creating easy-to-make, delicious, and healthy recipes. My recipes have been featured in RedBook Magazine, SheKnows.com, Examiner.com, and numerous others. I strongly believe that a healthy lifestyle starts with eating right, and that nothing is better than homemade meals.

I would love to connect with you, and discuss more healthy tips and share more recipes with you. You can find me through:

My website: **http://gourmetpersuasian.com/**
Email: **sharon@gourmetpersuasian.com**
Facebook: **https://www.facebook.com/gourmetpersuasian**
Twitter: **https://twitter.com/PersuAsianfood**
Instagram: **https://instagram.com/gourmetpersuasian/**
Pinterest: **https://www.pinterest.com/sharonchen0119/**
Google+: **https://plus.google.com/u/0/+SharonChen**